365
Everyday
Health Tips

365
Everyday
Health Tips

A Daily Guide to Improving

Health and Increasing Energy

Ottenheimer
PUBLISHERS, INC

Created and manufactured by Ottenheimer Publishers, Inc.
© 1996 Ottenheimer Publishers, Inc.
5 Park Center Court, Suite 300
Owings Mills, Maryland 21117, USA
Printed in the United States of America
SH120C

Note to the Reader

The information in *365 Everyday Health Tips* is designed to help increase your knowledge of traditional and alternative health information that may relieve health problems in some cases. This book is intended as a reference resource only, and does not purport to give medical advice. Do not use any remedy in this book without first consulting your physician or in place of prompt and proper medical care. The information contained in this book is not intended to substitute for the advice of your physician or any treatment that he or she may prescribe or recommend. Instead, use this book as a complement to your cooperative relationship with your physician.

Introduction

The United States is in the middle of a health care revolution. And the most important part of that revolution is not the federal government in Washington or the state and local governments where you live. Nor is it managed care and all the other changing aspects of the health marketplace.

The most important part of that revolution is you. It's you because only you can take control of your own health care by *learning to be responsible for your own health.*

Now I know that the word "responsibility" conjures up images of obligations and duties. But this is not what being responsible for your health really means. It means making rational decisions and using good judgment. And that's what the tips in this book are designed to help you do.

How?

The 365 suggestions you'll find here are simple, practical and easy-to-implement. Read a few of the tips, put down the book and put one of them into practice. It doesn't matter where you start or in which direction you head. The most recent research shows that making even small changes in your lifestyle will give you big pay-offs in health and vitality.

How do we know?

One of the most exciting aspects of health research today is that studies clearly demonstrate that *it is never too late* to start making small changes that will lead to big changes in how you feel. Even people who begin moderate exercise programs at the age of seventy, eighty or ninety achieve remarkable improvements in their physical, mental and spiritual health. And they begin to feel those benefits almost immediately.

The health research being done across the country also shows that *it is never too soon* to begin to take responsibility for your own health. The actions you take today will pay off not only immediately, for example, but also decades from now, because a healthier lifestyle gives you longer life.

What's more, you'll enjoy your later years more if you begin to take care of yourself now. Disease and severe physical decline are not natural parts of aging. And much of the memory loss, heart disease and adult-onset diabetes, and even some 60 percent of cancers, can be prevented.

You don't have to give up anything. In fact, if you substitute healthy pleasures—exercise, playful activity, healthy eating, love-making and travel, for example—for "pleasures" such as drinking, smoking, overeating and "vegging out" in front of the television, you will find that you have gained more than you could ever have imagined.

You probably know generally what to do but just need some help getting started. The simple, straightforward tips in this book can put you in the driver's seat and bring you improved health, increased vitality and, perhaps, even a happier life. Every day is a second chance. Take it and run.

Invest in your health now and "spend" that investment in your healthy years to come.

1. Buy American

Ask the produce manager in your supermarket where the produce you buy was grown.

Despite the fact that pesticides have been linked to cancer, nerve damage and birth defects, pesticide use has risen dramatically in recent years. And although you can't know what poison was used on what foods, you can minimize your risk.

In general, foods grown in the United States are exposed to lower levels of pesticides than foods grown outside this country. That's because the federal government regulates the amount of pesticide residues allowed in food.

In addition, some foods are safer than others. Corn, bananas, watermelon and cauliflower are less likely to be contaminated than lettuce, strawberries, celery, cherries and peaches because the husk and outer layers protect them from contamination.

You need five servings a day of fruits and vegetables to prevent cancer and other diseases. Try growing some of your own, rinse those that you buy and peel root vegetables such as potatoes, since pesticides can concentrate in their skins.

2. Break One Unhealthy Habit

Pick just one habit you want to eliminate and take the first step to break it this very minute. Research shows that it takes about three weeks to replace an unhealthy habit with a healthy one.

The first step is to identify the habit you want to change. The second step is to identify one healthy habit that will replace the unhealthy habit you're giving up. Go for a brisk forty-five-minute walk three times a week, for example, instead of stopping off for a few beers. Then identify the rewards you'll give yourself if you're successful in breaking the habit you've chosen.

Help yourself follow through with your plan by putting your commitment in writing.

3. Swim into Health

It's aerobic. It's great for flexibility. It strengthens almost every muscle, and it doesn't damage joints.

What is it?

Swimming—an activity in which, according to the American College of Sports Medicine, you can burn 360–750 calories an hour. (Compare this with 360–480 for aerobic dancing, 600 for jogging and 360–600 for calisthenics.) It strengthens your heart, builds muscular endurance and creates flexibility. And swimming is particularly helpful in preventing back pain and pain from sciatica and scoliosis.

Contact your local YMCA or health club for information about pool memberships. Some hotels even sell local pool memberships to make more regular use of their facilities.

If you decide to make swimming a part of your exercise routine, make sure there is a lifeguard on duty, wear protective goggles and always take a hot shower or bath when you're finished to rinse off the chlorine and other disinfectants.

4. Find the Best Doctor

Finding a good doctor with whom you can work is vital to your well-being. Yet many people put more effort into buying a car!

Unless you need a specialist for a chronic problem such as allergies, a general practitioner, family physician or primary care internist is frequently the best choice. That's because these doctors will have a broad spectrum of knowledge about a lot of different diseases and conditions. A "generalist" will frequently cost less than a specialist, as well!

First, get recommendations from friends and neighbors. Second, make an appointment for an initial consultation. Third, take a list of important questions with you. And fourth, find out where the physician went to school, if he or she is board-certified in a specialty, what hospitals the doctor is affiliated with and to which specialists and specialized medical centers patients are referred. You can frequently get a lot of information by reading the diplomas on waiting room walls.

And don't be afraid to discuss money. You should know the doctor's fees and what insurance coverage will be accepted.

But above all, trust your instincts. Is this someone you trust and feel comfortable with? Are patients kept waiting a long time? Does the doctor spend adequate time with you? The answers to these questions are not measures of your doctor's politeness. They're indicators of attitude toward patients. A doctor who con sistently overbooks patients so that people always have to wait— or, worse, never get enough time with the doctor to get their ques- tions answered—is someone who may be more interested in the bottom line than in your health.

5. Prevent a Heart Attack with Aspirin

Heart attack is still the leading cause of death for American men and women.

But results from the Harvard University Physicians' Health Study show that men over forty who have never had a heart attack and men of any age who have already had a heart attack can dramatically reduce their risk by taking a single tablet of aspirin every day. Women of all ages who have already had a heart attack may also benefit.

For women who have never had a heart attack, the picture is not as clear. The Harvard University Nurses' Health Study found that women who took six regular aspirin a week had a 30 percent lower risk of heart attack than those who did not, but more research is needed.

Although aspirin can greatly reduce the risk of a heart attack, because it thins the blood, it also may slightly increase the risk of a stroke. So before you start to use it on a regular basis, ask your doctor to help you weigh the pros and cons in light of your own health history.

6. Check Out Your Local Hospitals

Make sure that you know the strengths and weaknesses of your local hospitals before you need them. Find out what kinds of hospitals are in your area, their reputations and which ones your doctor is affiliated with. Check to see which ones your HMO or health plan has contracts with, and make sure that any hospital you might need to visit is accredited by the Joint Commission on Accreditation of Health Care Organizations.

For most ordinary medical problems, *community* or *general* hospitals are best because they are usually of small to medium size and are better able to give individual attention to patients. *Teaching* hospitals are usually affiliated with major medical schools, frequently have better access to the latest technology and are better for unusual or difficult medical problems. Some large medical centers specialize in treating one condition, such as cancer.

Don't wait until you need to go to a hospital to find out about it. Call the local American Hospital Association office or contact your state health department for information about specific hospitals in your area. And ask nurses, paramedics and other professional health workers in your community for recommendations.

7. Clean Out Your Medicine Cabinet

When was the last time you cleaned out your medicine cabinet? It's been a while, hasn't it?

Take the time to go through your medicine cabinet and get rid of prescription medications that are over one year old. Check the expiration dates on any over-the-counter products and throw out the ones that have expired. Then take any remaining medications and move them to a drawer or cabinet in another room. Medications can deteriorate in the heat and dampness of the bathroom.

And don't forget: Make sure that children cannot reach the place where medicines are stored.

8. Prepare for Battle

Make sure your medicine cabinet or closet has the supplies you need to handle any emergency.

A well-stocked medicine cabinet should have first-aid items such as sterile gauze pads and tape, sterile cotton balls, bandages for sprains, a hot water bottle or microwavable gel pack, a heating pad, surgical tweezers, a sterile needle and perhaps an anesthetic spray or antibiotic ointment. Over-the-counter pain relievers such as aspirin, acetaminophen and ibuprofen should be placed in another room, out of the bathroom's dampness. You may also want to stock a laxative, syrup of ipecac (for poisons that can be vomited up), charcoal (for poisons that can't), an antacid, a product to control diarrhea, a cough syrup or an expectorant, and over-the-counter nasal decongestants and antihistamines.

Take inventory of what's in your medicine cabinet now and make a list of what you need. A little preparation can save you a lot of time, trouble and worry. And don't forget to store everything out of a child's reach.

9. Laugh

Study after study indicates that every belly laugh boosts your immune system's disease fighters for a short period of time. So do your best to keep those immune system fighters at peak numbers by laughing as often as you can.

Today, hundreds of classic comedies are available to rent or buy. Cable movie and comedy channels can bring laughter into your home twenty-four hours a day, and many humorous tapes and CDs are also available.

10. Sin No More

Since 1965, Lester Breslow, M.D., has followed the health habits of 7,000 people in Alameda County, California. He has compiled a list of seven deadly health sins that have been linked with death at an early age. According to a report in the *New York Times*, the seven deadly health sins are:

1. Excessive alcohol consumption
2. Smoking
3. Obesity
4. Too much/too little sleep
5. Too little exercise
6. Snacking
7. Not eating breakfast

Are you guilty of any of these "health sins"? Mend your ways, and you will have more energy and live a longer, healthier life.

11. "Have a Nice Day"

Many people chuckle at the "Smile" button and its corny slogan, but a kind word or phrase may be more powerful than you imagine. A compliment, praise on the job or an enjoyable family gathering not only makes you feel good emotionally but also can boost your immune system for up to two days.

In a three-month study of 100 men, Arthur Stone, Ph.D., a psychologist at the State University of New York at Stony Brook, found that pleasant social activities and leisure activities such as jogging and fishing greatly improved the immune system. Dr. Stone also found that when the men experienced fewer pleasant daily events than usual, they became more susceptible to colds.

Researchers in Britain have reported findings similar to those of Dr. Stone.

So pin on that corny "Smile" button and make sure you tell those you encounter throughout the day just how great they are.

And don't be surprised if they begin to return the compliment.

12. Cut the Fat

One of the easiest ways to lose weight is by cutting down on dietary fat. The United States government recommends that the calories you get from fat be less than 30 percent of your total daily intake of calories. But cutting out the fat doesn't necessarily mean cutting out the fun.

If you like to snack on chips or nuts, for example, you don't have to give up snacking—just switch to pretzels. Or if you like to eat popcorn, eat only air-popped popcorn. At breakfast, eat plain whole-grain cereal instead of granola; have Canadian bacon instead of the fatty strips you grew up with. For dinner, try sirloin tip roast instead of steak. If you like fish, have water-packed instead of oil-packed canned fish. For dessert, try nonfat frozen yogurt or fat-free sorbet instead of ice cream.

13. Check Mole Changes with Your Doctor

The bad news is that skin cancer is the fastest-growing cancer in the United States today. Research shows that there are more than 500,000 new cases each year. People with fair skin, light hair and light eyes are at highest risk, but everybody must be careful about exposure to the sun. Cases of the deadliest form of skin cancer, melanoma, have grown by 1,500 percent in the past fifty years. Although melanoma accounts for only 5 percent of all skin cancer cases, it causes 75 percent of all skin cancer deaths.

The good news is that 90–95 percent of skin cancers are curable if detected early, and they can usually be removed in the doctor's office. Moles give clues to the early stages of skin cancer, so look for any changes in size, shape or color. Any changes should be checked by your doctor, as should any growth that itches or begins to bleed.

14. Launch an Offensive against Skin Cancer

What can you do to protect yourself from skin cancer?

According to Daniel Rigel, M.D., a doctor at the New York Hospital—Cornell Medical Center, there are five key strategies. One, learn to examine your own skin, using a full-length mirror and a handheld mirror to see your back. Don't forget to look at the soles of your feet and other hard-to-see parts of your body. Two, see a dermatologist if you notice a change in a skin mark or growth. This is a common early warning sign of skin cancer. Three, stay out of the sun between 10 A.M. and 2 P.M. (or between 11 A.M. and 3 P.M. during daylight saving time). Four, wear protective clothing and a hat. For every inch of rim on your hat, you will get a 10 percent decrease in skin cancer risk. And five, use sunscreens and sunblocks every day, year-round. Dr. Rigel recommends sunscreens of sun protection factor (SPF) 15 and higher. Make sure the sunscreen is waterproof and provides both UVA and UVB protection.

15. Reap What You Sow

Give something of yourself to others every day. Giving brings on what researchers call helper's high, a symptom of the "healthy-helping syndrome." According to Allan Luks and Peggy Payne, authors of *The Healing Power of Doing Good—The Health and Spiritual Benefits of Helping Others*, people who reach out to others experience greater overall health and well-being. You can benefit from helping others if you help frequently, help strangers and help without concern for rewards.

If you are thinking of volunteering your time to help others, *The Healing Power of Doing Good* may be just the place to start. The book contains information about more than seventy-five national organizations devoted to helping others.

16. Take a Walk

Walking strengthens your heart, lungs, muscles and bones. It relieves tension and increases energy. It doesn't cost anything, and it's safe. And for most people, the only equipment needed is a good pair of shoes.

Thirty minutes of walking can benefit you almost as much as more vigorous exercise does, experts at the Cooper Institute for Aerobics Research in Dallas report. And three ten-minute walks will help you as much as one thirty-minute walk. The latest research shows that the total amount of energy spent is what's important, not the intensity of the activity. Either walking or running that uses up 300 calories will bring you just about the same health benefits.

Women who walk a mile a day can delay bone loss, and women who begin a walking program during or after menopause can even reverse the rapid bone loss common at this time, according to scientists at the U.S. Department of Agriculture.

So put on your walking shoes and head outdoors. Or if the weather is bad, take a few laps at the local mall. Some malls even sponsor early-bird walking programs. If your mall doesn't have one, why not start one yourself?

17. Women: Check Your Breasts

Women should begin monthly breast self-examination at age twenty and continue it throughout life, experts suggest. Eighty percent of cancerous tumors are discovered by women themselves.

How should you examine your breasts? At first, you may want to examine them daily, to get used to how your breasts normally feel. Over time, you'll be able to notice normal changes. Then every month, a few days after your period, stand in front of a mirror with your arms at your sides. Look for puckering or dimpling and changes in breast size, coloring and texture. Raise your arms above your head and look again. Then gently squeeze your nipples and look for any discharge.

When you get in the shower, raise one arm and, with fingers held flat, gently feel about your breast for lumps or thickening. Use your right hand to examine your left breast and your left hand to examine your right breast.

Then lie down, place a pillow under your right shoulder and put your right hand behind your head. Starting at the outermost top edge of your right breast, slowly move your flat fingers in a spiraling motion toward the nipple, examining the whole breast. Feel for lumps from under your armpit all the way to your collarbone. Repeat this procedure with your left breast.

18. Men: Check Your Testicles

Testicular self-examination saves lives. That's because although testicular cancer is common in men between fifteen and thirty-five years of age, the cure rate is very high—95 to 97 percent—when the cancer is detected early.

Men under age thirty-five should examine their testes once a month. After a warm bath or shower, when the skin around the scrotum is relaxed, gently roll each testicle in both hands. If you feel a hard or unusual lump, see your doctor as soon as possible to determine if it is benign.

19. Cut Down on Caffeine

If you drink more than one cup of coffee a day, you could be hooked on the most widely used drug in the world: caffeine.

Caffeine takes effect in about thirty minutes and lasts from two to eight hours. It stimulates alertness chemicals in the brain, and that perks you up. But it also raises insulin levels, and that brings you down. Irritability, nervousness, insomnia and increased blood pressure can all result from 300 milligrams of caffeine—about the amount contained in three five-ounce cups of coffee or six twelve-ounce cans of soda.

In addition, there are a number of relaxation techniques—deep breathing, for example—that you can use to help you relax without a caffeinated drink in hand. A good starting point for learning these techniques is to read *The Relaxation Response* and *Beyond the Relaxation Response* by Harvard Medical School professor Herbert Benson, M.D.

20. Beat Caffeine without Withdrawal

If you're trying to cut back on your caffeine intake, don't quit cold turkey. Taper off slowly or you may develop severe headaches, depression, fatigue and the inability to concentrate. If you stop suddenly, expect a painful headache about eighteen hours after your last cup of coffee. A gentler route is to gradually cut down on your caffeine intake over the next four to five weeks.

Researchers at Johns Hopkins University School of Medicine have shown that caffeine produces a druglike dependency. This means that you can develop a tolerance to the "drug," then suffer withdrawal symptoms if you stop abruptly. To avoid this problem, cut back on your caffeine by about 20 percent a week. You may want to substitute herbal teas or drinks made from chicory or ground roasted barley, wheat or chestnut. Or you can switch to decaffeinated coffee and sodas.

21. Know Your Caffeine Count

If you want to cut back on caffeine, you need to know how much you're taking in. Caffeine occurs naturally in coffee, tea and chocolate. It also occurs unnaturally—as an added ingredient—in many soft drinks and even in some medications. Listed on the following page are the caffeine contents of popular beverages.

Brewed coffee: 110–150 mg per 5-oz cup
Instant coffee: 40–108 mg per 5-oz cup
Hot Tea: 20–50 mg per 5-oz cup
Iced tea: 22–36 mg per 12-oz serving
Hot cocoa: 2–8 mg per 6-oz cup
Coca-Cola: 45.6 mg per 12-oz serving
Pepsi-Cola: 38.4 mg per 12-oz serving
Jolt: 72 mg per 12-oz serving

Most adults can tolerate three cups of coffee, or 300 milligrams of caffeine a day without experiencing "the jitters" and other reactions. Now if you want to cut back on your caffeine intake, you know where you stand.

22. Make Sure the Shoe Fits before You Wear It

A good exercise shoe must support your foot where it needs support and provide flexibility where your foot bends.

Before you purchase a pair of shoes, take one, grasp the shoe at the front and back, and bend it. If the shoe bends in the middle, it will probably not give you the support you need. If the shoe bends at the ball of your foot, it will.

Everyone's feet are different, and individual forms of exercise require specific types of shoes. Explain to the salesperson what type of exercise you will be doing and ask for his or her recommendation. Try on several different pairs.

If the shoe fits, you will be able to wear it in good health.

23. Try a Water Workout

Instead of running in the park or working out in the gym or health club, try jogging in your local pool—especially if you are overweight, recovering from an injury or pregnant. An aerobic exercise such as running can put a lot of stress on muscles and joints when performed on land, but water cushions and protects the body.

If you work out in water, check the pool's thermometer to make sure the water temperature is between eighty-two and eighty-six degrees Fahrenheit. If the water is too cold, you may feel pain in your muscles. If it's too warm, you may feel weak or even faint. Check with your doctor before beginning a water program if you have a heart condition or high blood pressure.

24. Make Your Beef Trim and Lean

Beef is much leaner today than it was twenty or thirty years ago, but it still has so much artery-clogging fat that you need to be selective.

The fattiest cut of beef is, unfortunately, the one that sounds most desirable: "Prime." The next grade of meat, "Choice," has about 40 percent less fat than Prime. "Select" beef has 20 percent less fat than Choice.

It isn't only the grade—Prime, Choice or Select—that counts, though. The cut of beef counts as well. The leanest cuts are sirloin tip, top round and London broil.

Remember to trim all fat from the meat before cooking and to eat only three- to four-ounce portions.

25. Pop a Potato into the Micro

When you have the "hungries," treat yourself to a belly-filling potato instead of a pile of potato chips. Potatoes are extremely nutritious and low in fat, and one potato has only 200 calories! Research has shown that potatoes are also rich in B vitamins, potassium and iron. They are also fair sources of fiber and protein and provide half of your daily requirement of vitamin C.

So the next time you're in the mood for a snack, grab a potato, wash it, pierce its skin with a fork and pop it into the microwave. In less than ten minutes, you'll have a healthy treat.

Then top it with a full-flavored salsa or smooth nonfat yogurt. You'll be surprised at how delicious it tastes!

26. Get Your Calcium the Natural Way

Are you concerned about getting enough calcium?

If you don't want to take dietary supplements, consider getting your calcium the old-fashioned way: through food!

Nutritional research shows that we require the following amounts of calcium at these ages:

1–11 years: 800 milligrams a day
11–24 years: 1,200 milligrams a day
25 and older: 800 milligrams a day

Some nutrition experts believe that postmenopausal women need 1,200–1,500 milligrams of calcium a day because of their greater risk of developing osteoporosis. Pregnant women may also need more to meet the demands of a developing fetus.

You may want to avoid the best sources of calcium—dairy products—because of their high fat content. But skim milk, low-fat cheese and nonfat yogurt have just as much calcium as their high-fat cousins.

Other foods that provide good amounts of calcium include tofu, soybeans, almonds, figs, canned salmon or sardines, broccoli, spinach and kale.

With such a wide variety of sources, you should have no difficulty getting your calcium naturally.

27. Make a Healthier Gravy

If a delicious gravy is the highlight of some meals for you, you may not have to give it up, even though it's super-saturated with fat. That's because an inexpensive device called a gravy separator can literally separate the fat from the meat's juices.

Pick one up from your local supermarket, cook your favorite meat, then pour the juice from the pan into the separator and let it stand for a few minutes. Most of the fat will gradually rise to the top. You can then retrieve the juices and leave the fat behind.

You can achieve the same effect by refrigerating any gravies or sauces you make. As before, the fat will rise. The fat will congeal at cool temperatures, and then you can easily remove it.

In either case, you can have your gravy and eat healthily, too!

28. Practice Kitchen Caution

Bacteria, viruses, molds and yeasts in food cause as many as fifty million cases of food poisoning in the United States each year. You can keep this from happening to you and your family by following these simple suggestions.

- Always use a fresh kitchen towel when cooking.
- Don't allow pets to get near your food.
- Don't keep food at room temperature for more than sixty minutes—before or after cooking.
- When marinating poultry and other meats, do so only in the refrigerator.
- Don't reuse marinade without first bringing it to a boil.
- Keep stuffing separate from the turkey or chicken in which it was cooked.

29. Slash the Fat in Salad Dressing

The majority of salad dressings available in the supermarket contain high levels of fat. In fact, some dressings get as much as 90 *percent* of their calories from fat—nearly three times the amount they should! But you can avoid that problem by making your own healthy low-fat salad dressings.

There are many different recipes for healthy salad dressings. As a general rule, use one-third less oil and one-third more vinegar if you are making a vinaigrette dressing. For a healthy creamy dressing, substitute plain nonfat yogurt for fattier dairy products, then spice it up with a mixture of onion, dill, garlic, basil, oregano and pepper.

30. Bet on Beta-Carotene

Study after study indicates that foods rich in beta-carotene and its other carotenoid brethren—luetin and lycopene, for example—help your body's cancer-fighting systems reach their maximum efficiency.

How much do you need?

Although more research is necessary to answer that question, most scientists seem to feel that half of a cantaloupe, a couple of carrots or a sweet potato once a day can probably do the job. Other foods that are rich in beta-carotene include mangoes, kale and watercress. In general, dark green, orange and yellow fruits and vegetables are good sources of this vital nutrient.

31. Reduce the Fat in the Meat You Eat

You can hardly read about nutrition, diet or cooking without being reminded of the importance of reducing fat in your diet. But for many people, a meal is not really a meal unless it includes meat. And many meats are high in fat.

What can you do?

Nutritional experts generally agree that your total fat intake should not come to more than 30 percent of your total daily calories. You can still eat meat regularly—a couple of times a week—and meet the nutritional recommendations concerning dietary fat if you do the following:

- Trim all obvious fat.
- Choose only lean cuts.
- Avoid frying meat.
- Bake or broil meat.
- Keep portions to three to four ounces.

32. Become a Part-Time Vegetarian

Most of us know that the traditional American diet of meat and potatoes, with a heavy commitment to butter and other dairy products, is not a healthy way to eat. But few of us can imagine life as a true vegetarian.

Yet nutritional experts generally agree that the vegetarian's low-fat, high-fiber diet reduces the risk of heart disease, lowers cholesterol levels, lowers blood pressure and stimulates better digestion.

If you can't give up meat entirely, all is not lost. Asian cuisine, for example, when lightly stir-fried in chicken broth rather than oil, is a healthy mix of vegetables and meats. And many other ethnic cuisines offer the same approach.

Make vegetables, grains, legumes and fruits a major part of your daily diet, and you can still enjoy a steak—and even dairy products—once in a while.

33. Watch Out for Unhealthy "Health Foods"

There are healthy foods, and then there are foods that are advertised as "health foods" but are actually about as unhealthy as you can get.

Many people believe they are eating a healthier breakfast when they switch from a boxed cereal to homemade "natural" granola, for example. But a brand-name or generic box of shredded wheat breakfast cereal is usually high in fiber and low in fat and sodium, while granola is generally high in fat and calories.

Bran is another example. It's healthy by itself. But throw it into a muffin with lots of oil, and a bran muffin may contain far more fat than it does fiber.

Always read the labels and check the ingredients in the foods you buy. Boycott those with fats, oils and sugars listed near the beginning of the ingredients list. The name of the product may sound healthy, but the product itself may be a nutritional nightmare.

34. Avoid "Guaranteed" Weight Loss Plans

Are you considering a diet plan that "absolutely guarantees" that you'll lose weight quickly and easily?

Are you tempted to start a weight loss plan that is based on a new miracle food or drink that will help you lose a lot of weight in a short period of time? If you answered yes to either question, please think again.

Why? Because the diet won't work. Decades of research at centers all across the country have shown that there are two key factors in any successful weight loss plan: (1) You need to evaluate your eating habits and make permanent changes, and (2) you need to develop a program of regular moderate aerobic exercise that works for you. Any other approach generally means you'll lose weight initially, then gain back more than you lost.

35. Buy Fresh Foods

If you buy mainly processed foods, rethink your shopping habits. Processing generally destroys vitamins and other valuable nutrients. That's why fresh vegetables are generally better nutrition bargains than frozen or canned vegetables. And they frequently cost less, too.

If you must buy processed foods, buy frozen rather than canned. Freezing destroys far fewer nutrients than canning.

36. Be Creative in the Kitchen

Do you sometimes find that you know what you should do but you don't know how to do it? You may want to eat less fat or sugar, for example, but find that your favorite recipes call for sugar or eggs.

Remember, it's not all or nothing when it comes to eating healthy. So be creative and experiment. If you normally use sugar when you make corn bread or muffins, use only half of the amount your recipe calls for. Or if your recipe calls for one egg, substitute two egg whites in its place. Give it a try—you probably won't even notice the change!

37. Listen to Your Children

Most people can remember some hard times from their youth, but today there are even more sources of stress for even younger children: 50 percent of marriages end in divorce; both parents often work; alcohol, drugs and cigarettes are more readily available; and the pressure from peers to engage in sexual activity is significant.

Besides creating unhappy children, stressful conditions can result in physical illness or emotional problems. One of the most important things you can do to prevent this is to encourage a child to express his or her feelings. Communicate with your child from the earliest years on, and you can not only prevent many problems but also greatly minimize those that do occur.

38. Get to the Bottom of Lower Back Pain

About seventy-five million Americans suffer from lower back pain at some point in their lives, and more often than not, the cause is unknown.

Research has shown that most common backaches respond to bed rest on a firm mattress, an over-the-counter pain reliever and a heating pad or ice. But if your doctor has ruled out all of the major physical causes of lower back pain, stress may be the problem. So the next time your back goes out, try to identify the situations in your life that may be causing stress and triggering pain.

When you become aware of which stressful events are troubling you, it will be possible to eliminate them. And even if you can't totally leave them behind, sometimes just acknowledging them is enough to reduce their impact on your emotional life—and on your back.

39. Don't Worry

Worrying prevents you from enjoying life without helping you find real solutions to your troubles. And it causes your endocrine glands to release hormones that can interfere with your digestion and cause an upset stomach.

You can reduce the physical effects of worry by creating a positive mental image to block it. If you have a job interview, for example, imagine yourself at the interview calm and confident. Picture yourself as just the person for the job. Envision the interviewer smiling and impressed with you and your responses. Feel the warm, confident sensations that these images bring about.

40. Save Your Skin from Stress

We turn red with embarrassment and white with fear. The skin, the largest organ of the human body, reflects all our emotions and can suffer because of them. Hives, itching, eczema, rashes and psoriasis may be brought on or aggravated by stress.

When your skin breaks out, take a moment to sit quietly and ask yourself how you are really feeling. Are you angry? Do you feel there is too much pressure at work or at home? Do you feel guilty?

If you answer yes to any of these questions, and if your doctor determines that your skin problems are not caused by an infection, allergy or disease, regular practice of a relaxation technique may reduce stress and help keep your skin blemish-free. Ask your doctor for information about meditation, yoga, biofeedback and other methods that may help.

41. Take It Easy

If you are impatient, competitive and hard on yourself (and maybe on others as well), it probably isn't easy for you to take it easy. But it may be the healthiest thing for you to do.

Medical research has shown that stress (your body's chemical response to certain life situations) can contribute to some forms of cardiovascular disease and make you "coronary-prone." Stressors—situations that trigger stress—raise blood pressure, heart rate, blood flow and metabolism rate. If stressors provoke these physiological changes too frequently and too strongly, many doctors believe they can lead to heart disease.

At Stanford University School of Medicine, patients were taught a simple relaxation technique that helped them significantly reduce their blood pressure. While they imagined a tranquil scene, they tensed and then relaxed their muscles. The patients practicing this technique lowered their blood pressure twice as much as the patients who received medical treatment but no instruction in relaxation techniques.

If you find yourself reacting strongly to everyday events and having a hard time relaxing, talk to your doctor about some relaxation techniques you can learn to help you take it easy.

42. Avoid Precut Vegetables

How many times have you been in a hurry and bought precut vegetables in plastic bags at the supermarket? According to the *New York Times*, you may save time, but you probably lose nutritional benefits by purchasing precut products.

All precut vegetables need to be kept in cold temperatures. This is essential to preserving the food's quality. Many stores do not do this properly—or at all.

If you must buy precut vegetables, check the "use by" date on the package. Foods lose vitamins over time. The fresher the product, the higher the nutritional value of the food. If there is no "use by" date on the package, don't buy the product.

43. Benefit from Vitamin E

Recent newspaper headlines and broadcast reports may have led you to consider taking vitamin E to help fight cancer, heart disease or premature aging. Be aware, however, that the final word on vitamin E is not yet in.

Most researchers studying vitamin E are taking it themselves, although many are not yet recommending it to the public.

Why not? That's hard to answer, but some scientists feel they don't have enough proof that vitamin E is as safe and effective as it appears.

Vitamin E is usually sold in gelcaps in doses ranging from 100 to 1,000 international units (IUs). Studies indicate that you will probably get the most benefit from taking 400 IUs daily.

Check with your doctor before taking vitamin E because it can affect the time it takes your blood to clot.

44. Get Help for von Willebrand's Disease

Get help for von what? Von Willebrand's disease is an inherited clotting disorder like hemophilia that is unknown to most people—including 90 percent of those who have it! Yet it can affect 1 in 100 men and women.

The disease is not life-threatening, but it does cause frequent nosebleeds, bleeding gums, easy bruising and excessive menstrual flow. A blood test is now available to diagnose the disease. The test is recommended for any adolescent girl or woman with heavy menstrual periods for which there is no obvious cause and for people with frequent, unexplained nosebleeds or bruising.

Fortunately, a new treatment is now available—a prescription drug called desmopressin acetate—so if you have any of the symptoms associated with von Willebrand's disease, consult your doctor.

45. Know the Signs of Mountain Sickness

You know all about motion sickness and morning sickness, but have you ever heard of mountain sickness?

Although not much is known about this condition, some researchers believe that less oxygen reaches the brain at high altitudes, which may impair the part of the brain involved with speech and making judgments. As a result, many people get confused and make dangerous mistakes. They may also get headaches and vomit.

Everyone who travels to the mountains should be concerned about mountain sickness. Faulty judgments at high altitudes can result in going too near the edge of a cliff or ignoring the risks of an avalanche.

If you find yourself acting "funny," it may be time to head back down to the valley.

46. Treat Your Children Well

If your child is among the 25 percent of American children who are not protected against common childhood diseases, make an appointment with your pediatrician or a health clinic today.

Many parents do not know when their children should get recommended inoculations and when they should get booster shots. The federal Centers for Disease Control and Prevention recommends the following schedule for childhood vaccinations:

Birth–2 months:	hepatitis B
2 months:	polio; diphtheria, tetanus, pertussis (DTP); *Haemophilus influenzae* type B (HiB)
2–4 months:	hepatitis B
4 months:	polio, DTP, HiB
6 months:	DTP, HiB
6–18 months:	hepatitis B, polio
12–15 months:	HiB; measles, mumps, rubella (MMR)

```
12–18 months:   chicken pox, DTP
   4–6 years:   polio, DTP, MMR
```
Talk to your doctor about what vaccinations your child needs and when. Since some vaccines are prepared in eggs, make sure your doctor knows if your child is allergic to eggs.

47. Try Tofu

Tofu has been an important part of the Asian diet for centuries. In America, however, this fresh, white soybean curd has been a favorite of health food devotees for only the past twenty-five years. Yet there is new evidence to suggest that all of us may want to add tofu to our diets.

A recent study in the *New England Journal of Medicine* revealed that eating three to four ounces of soybeans daily reduces cholesterol levels—and that the higher the level of cholesterol, the greater the reduction! And other research suggests that the soybeans in tofu may also help prevent cancer and osteoporosis.

Be careful when purchasing tofu. Unpackaged tofu stored in water can contain harmful bacteria. Don't buy it. Buy tofu only in sealed packages and cook it in your oven at a temperature above 160 degrees Fahrenheit to kill any harmful bacteria. Tofu can easily be mixed into sauces and casseroles. It has little flavor of its own and assumes the flavors of other spices you use. It's also a great source of protein.

48. Use Antibiotics Only for Bacterial Infections

There has been a dramatic increase in bacteria that are resistant to antibiotics. As a result, these bacteria can cause serious and sometimes fatal diseases such as pneumonia and meningitis.

Researchers from Barcelona to Atlanta have reported that the rise in antibiotic-resistant bacteria is due to the inappropriate use of antibiotics. They have found that instead of being prescribed exclusively for bacterial infections, the drugs are being handed out to treat cold viruses as well—even though antibiotics are useless against viruses.

The result? Less than ten years ago, penicillin-resistant bacteria were found in only 0.02 percent of people studied. Today, 25 percent of adults studied had infections resistant to penicillin; in children under age six, 41 percent of infections were resistant to penicillin.

The next time your doctor prescribes antibiotics, ask if they're really necessary. Chicken soup may be better!

49. Get a Vaccination before Your Vacation

If you are one of the twenty-four million Americans who travel abroad each year, you may want to consider getting a shot to protect yourself against hepatitis A. Hepatitis A is a viral inflammation of the liver. It is spread through contaminated food and water as well as through close person-to-person contact with an infected individual.

The Centers for Disease Control and Prevention has recently released this recommendation for travelers: If you are traveling to Mexico, Central America, South America, the Caribbean, Southern Europe, Asia or Africa, you should consider getting a Hepatitis A vaccination.

For a free booklet on traveler's health information, you can call the Centers for Disease Control Information Hotline, which provides recorded information by phone or written information by fax, at 404-332-4559.

50. Get a Good Night's Sleep

If you occasionally have trouble sleeping, here are five surefire strategies to knock you out.

First, learn to associate your bed with rest, quiet and sleep.

Don't eat in bed or take work to bed.

Second, make your bedroom comfortable and conducive to sleep. Keep the temperature at around sixty-eight degrees Fahrenheit and make sure your mattress is comfortable.

Third, stick to a regular sleep schedule. During the workweek and on weekends, go to sleep at the same time and wake up at the same time.

Fourth, if you can't fall asleep soon after going to bed, get up and leave the bedroom. Read or watch a little TV, but don't do it in your bedroom.

Fifth, avoid alcohol, caffeine and exercise late in the day. They all interfere with sleep.

If you follow these tips, occasional insomnia should trouble you no more. But see a doctor if insomnia persists.

51. Put Your Best Foot Forward

If you're not wearing the right shoes, that pain in your back that won't go away may be originating in your feet.

Researchers in Israel have found that flexible, soft-soled shoes with shock-absorbing cushions significantly reduce pain for many people. Cushioning shoe inserts can also be of great help.

So put your best foot forward and kiss that nagging backache good-bye!

52. Soothe an Upset Stomach with Chamomile

There are many products available over the counter to treat digestive problems, and more products are appearing on the market all the time. These products, however, vary greatly in their effectiveness and may even produce some unacceptable side effects of their own.

Chamomile is an herb that is widely used in Europe for digestive disorders. It is effective at settling an upset stomach and has shown no toxic effects. (Rarely, however, someone may be allergic to the herb.)

The next time you experience indigestion, steep one-half ounce of chamomile in one and one-half cups of boiling water for ten minutes. This will produce a strong chamomile tea. You can soothe and settle your stomach naturally by drinking the tea throughout the day as needed. You can buy chamomile tea bags in most supermarkets, or you can order loose chamomile tea leaves from companies such as American Health Food in Tucson, Arizona. Call 1-800-858-2143 for information.

53. Kill Bathroom Germs without Toxic Cleansers

We all know that the bathroom can be a major source of infection, and we try to keep it as germ-free as possible. What many of us do not realize, however, is that many of the bathroom disinfectants on the market contain toxic ingredients that can be absorbed through the skin—or even cause skin burns.

Check the ingredients in your bathroom disinfectants and avoid products containing phenol and cresol. If these corrosive chemicals are absorbed by your body, they can cause nausea, paralysis, coma, even death. Simply because they are readily available in stores does not mean they are safe.

Keep your bathroom germ-free by using safe alternatives such as detergents, baking soda, antibacterial soaps or rubbing alcohol.

54. Use Natural Oven Cleaners

Many commercial oven cleaners certainly dissolve grease, but they can also cause chemical burns that practically dissolve your skin, too.

Instead of using these highly corrosive cleaners, scour your oven with baking soda. Put one-quarter cup of ammonia in the closed oven overnight to loosen the grease before you scrub with the baking soda.

While it may seem easier to buy one of the many products available at the supermarket, it may not be the healthy thing to do. Many researchers have linked common cleaners with a wide variety of health problems, from headaches to brain damage.

55. Repel Moths with Cedar or Herbs

Was that a moth you just saw? Don't go for the mothballs to protect your good woolen clothing. Some of the chemicals in mothballs may be carcinogenic. Research has shown that the ingredients in mothballs give off a vapor that can irritate the skin, eyes and throat. The fumes can sometimes cause nausea, headaches and even anemia and seizures.

To protect yourself and your fine woolens, try a more natural moth repellent such as cedar chips or cedar blocks soaked in real cedar oil. Or, use a sachet of dried tobacco, lavender and whole peppercorns, or a mixture of rosemary and mint.

56. Get the Radon Out

You can't see it, smell it or taste it, but radon can kill. It is a naturally occurring radioactive gas, primarily from decaying rock formations under basement floors, that affects millions of homes all across the United States. Radon is the leading cause of lung cancer among nonsmokers, killing as many as 30,000 people a year, according to the National Cancer Institute.

You can test your home for as little as ten to twenty-five dollars with an easy-to-use kit. Look in the phone book under "Radon" to find a store near you that sells these kits. If you find high radon levels (the tester should include details about radon levels), perform the test a second time to be sure.

You can rid your home of radon on a short-term basis by opening all basement windows for maximum cross-ventilation. For a more long-lasting solution, seal any basement cracks and openings, including drains. If radon levels remain high, check the phone book for a professional radon service company that can further seal your home and install a special ventilation system.

57. Run a Bathroom Safety Check

While it may get you squeaky clean, water can also be hazardous to your health. To keep everyone in your family—from children to senior citizens—safe, attach securely fastened grab bars in bathtubs and in shower stalls to prevent falls, and make sure to put a nonslip surface or rubber mat with suction cups on the bottom of each tub and shower. Remove any electrical appliances to another room or swap them for battery-operated models.

Also, don't forget that all bathroom rugs should have rubberized backings to keep them—and you—from sliding!

58. Reduce the Odds of a Kitchen Fire

If you're like many people, you probably enjoy sitting at the kitchen table, either for a quiet moment alone or to enjoy lively conversation with family and friends. But don't forget that this warm and cozy room also has potential hazards.

To increase the safety of your kitchen, remember these four rules: One, keep window curtains away from the range, where a breeze can blow them over a burner. Two, wear close-fitting clothing when working in the kitchen—especially when you're using a burner—so sleeves don't catch fire. Three, if a grease fire starts in the oven, close the oven door and turn off the heat. And four, if a grease fire starts in a pan on a burner, turn off the burner and cover the pan.

59. Run a Safety Check on Your Garage

Many of us rarely think about a garage except as a place to store junk, park the car or hold a sale. But a garage can pose a few hazards to the unwary. Here are a few things you should specifically look for.

- Tools should be properly stored, and flammable liquids and materials need to be vented and stored according to the manufacturer's instructions.
- If you have a garage door that opens automatically, make sure that the controls are out of the reach of children. A child could be caught under a closing door, and older models do not have a safety feature that will stop or reverse the door if it senses an obstacle.
- If your garage door opens manually and folds in sections, make sure there are handles on each section to avoid injuring fingers.

60. Pay Attention to Floor Safety

Most people feel secure and safe at home. Yet nearly 20,000 people are killed in home accidents each year, and millions suffer serious injuries.

Many of these tragic accidents are falls, yet falls are easily prevented. Keep any rugs smooth—even a small wrinkle can cause someone to trip. And if you notice that the corners of the carpeting are curling, secure them with carpet tape.

Never run electrical wires under the carpeting. Electrical cords can dry out or fray and need replacement. You can't see what condition they're in when they're hidden under carpeting. Also, don't run wires across "lanes" where people walk.

The fall you prevent might be your own!

61. Reach Out and Touch Someone

A hug may be just as important to your health as good food and lots of exercise.

Researchers at Johns Hopkins University School of Medicine found that when people were touched, their heartbeats slowed. One physician found that routine pulse-taking completely suppressed irregular heartbeats in a study of 300 coronary care patients.

If the human connection is that powerful, think what a hug, a pat on the back or even a handshake will do!

62. Cherish Your Friends

Studies show that from the most primitive to the most developed societies, friendship has a protective, positive effect on people. In fact, friends can even help keep each other healthy.

A study of 7,000 people in Alameda County, California, has revealed that people with more social contacts outlive people with fewer contacts.

Why? No one knows for sure. But researchers at the University of Alabama have found that people who have close friendships have lower blood pressure and suffer from less heart disease and depression than people who don't. And studies at Duke University show that friends act as loving buffers against the damaging effects of stress.

Cherish your friends. Reach out to others in friendship.

63. Fight Aging with Antioxidants

Free radicals are chemical molecules that can harm your health and accelerate aging. Research has shown that certain foods contain antioxidants, which help your body defend itself against free radicals. These antioxidants—beta-carotene, vitamins C and E, plus the mineral selenium—can easily be increased in your diet by increasing your consumption of fruits, nuts and vegetables.

Beta-carotene is found in asparagus, broccoli, cantaloupe, carrots, dried apricots, green beans, peaches, spinach, sweet potatoes and tomato juice.

Vitamin C is found in broccoli, brussels sprouts, cantaloupe, grapefruit juice, green peppers, orange juice, oranges and papaya.

Vitamin E is found in almonds, hazelnuts, pecans, raw wheat germ, sunflower seed oil, sunflower seeds and wheat germ oil.

Selenium is found in broccoli, cabbage, onions, seafood and whole-grain cereals and breads.

Keep in mind that the fresher the food and the less heat to which it is exposed, the higher its nutrient content.

64. Smother That Glow

If the threat of lung cancer hasn't yet convinced you to give up smoking, perhaps this will: The average smoker receives a yearly dose of radiation from cigarettes that is equal to 250–300 chest X rays, according to a California physician who wrote to the medical journal *Lancet*.

The source? Tobacco growers use high-phosphate fertilizers, which are natural sources of radioactive polonium. The radioactive nuclides from this material are carried in the smoke to your lungs.

Think about it. As you sit in the dark at night, smoking a cigarette with radioactive material in it, your cigarette may not be the only thing in the room that's glowing! Call your local chapter of the American Cancer Society today and ask for information about their smoking cessation programs.

65. Don't Drink and Walk

Drunk-driving deaths have declined in the past fifteen years, since the national conscience was stirred by groups such as Mothers Against Drunk Driving (MADD). While many people are not drinking and driving, too many people who have had too much to drink are walking home. And it is their last walk.

A recent Centers for Disease Control and Prevention/National Highway Traffic Safety Administration study revealed that 36 percent of the pedestrians over age fourteen killed by cars were legally drunk. In fact, pedestrians who are drunk account for 14 percent of all vehicle-related deaths, regardless of their age.

While walking is good for most people, and a little moderate drinking may be good for some, walking and drinking is not a good idea for anyone.

If you've had too much to drink, call a sober friend for a ride.

66. Lay Down Your Arms

The right to own a gun is a hot topic in politics. But the right thing in politics may be the wrong thing for your health and the health of your family.

Public health researchers looked at 444 murders in three counties in Washington State, Tennessee and Ohio. All the murders occurred in the victims' homes. Half of the victims were killed by gunshots, and the guns were ones that the victims kept in their homes for protection. The researchers also found that 77 percent of the victims were killed by someone they knew; half were killed in arguments or because of a love triangle. Only 3.6 percent were killed by unknown intruders.

Heavy drinking, drug abuse and domestic violence greatly increased the chances of being murdered at home.

67. Use Garlic to Lower Cholesterol

Who would have guessed that the favorite ingredient in Italian cuisine and the preferred method for keeping vampires away could also help you stay healthy? According to more than a dozen recent studies, you can reduce cholesterol levels by eating garlic.

Researchers at New York Medical College reported that total cholesterol levels were lowered by 9 percent when small amounts of garlic—one-half to one clove a day—were added to the diet.

68. Get Moving

Adults over age sixty-five who are physically active are up to 66 percent more likely to live long lives than their peers who are not active.

Researchers studied 1,874 men and women in Boston, 1,488 in New Haven, Connecticut, and 1,815 in two Iowa counties. According to the results of the studies, published in the *American Journal of Public Health*, overall mortality during the study period was 50 to 66 percent lower in the more physically active groups than in the less active groups. Adults who were active also suffered less physical impairment. The activities studied—walking, for example—were not strenuous, and well within the reach of most people.

So when you get up in the morning, don't just sit down and smell the coffee. Go out for a walk, enjoy the sunshine and smell the flowers.

69. Run for Your Life

Add some hard-breathing aerobic exercise to your life and help slow down a part of aging that affects even the healthiest people: stiffening of the arteries.

Researchers tested the aerobic capacity of 146 men and women between the ages of twenty-one and ninety-six who had no trace of cardiovascular disease. And they found that, even in this healthy group, arterial stiffness was two to five times higher at age ninety than at age twenty.

When researchers compared fourteen men over age fifty-four who competed regularly in distance running with nonathletes of the same age, however, they found that arterial stiffness was up to 35 percent lower in the men who engaged in aerobic exercise.

The results, which were reported in the journal *Circulation*, show that regular aerobic exercise can reduce the arterial stiffness—a condition that sets the stage for heart disease—that comes naturally with aging.

70. Use RICE for Strains and Sprains

Even though a sports injury may require a doctor's attention, there *are* things you can do immediately. What you need first is RICE: rest, ice, compression and elevation.

First, sit down and rest the injured area, so you don't increase the pain and swelling or do further damage. Second, use a bag of crushed ice to prevent or reduce swelling. Apply the ice for fifteen to twenty minutes every two hours. *Never* sleep with ice on the injury. If you have an injured foot, ankle or hand, you can immerse it in ice water (no colder than sixty degrees Fahrenheit) for fifteen minutes at a time rather than applying crushed ice.

Third, use an elastic wrap bandage to compress and support the injured area. Don't wrap too tightly. And fourth, if at all possible, elevate the injured area with a pillow to help reduce swelling and ensure proper blood flow. Elevate your legs twenty-eight to thirty inches. Be on your back as much as possible.

If pain persists after forty-eight hours, see your doctor.

71. Leave the Driving to Others

As hard as it may be to admit, there comes a time when a senior citizen should park his or her car for good. Accident rates skyrocket in people over seventy-five, and those over eighty are as dangerous on the road as teenagers. What's more, according to the *Wall Street Journal*, a senior citizen is less likely to survive an accident, even when wearing a seat belt.

Ask your ophthalmologist or family physician if he or she thinks you still have the sharp eyes and quick reflexes necessary to drive.

Depending on what your physician finds, it may be fine to continue driving, or you may want to restrict your driving to daytime trips within your neighborhood—just as you probably restricted your teenager during his accident-prone years. Or it may even be time to hang up your car keys for good.

72. Try a Little Exercise for a Lot of Benefit

If you have mild to moderately high blood pressure, a mild to moderate exercise program may be just what you need.

The American College of Sports Medicine reviewed more than forty studies on the effects of endurance exercise on high blood pressure. The study concluded that exercise at a less than peak level may lower blood pressure as much as or even more than more strenuous exercise.

This is good news for those who may not be in shape for high-intensity exercise. Ask your doctor to help you design an exercise program that meets your needs.

73. Minimize Arthritis Pain with Plain Old Aspirin

The pharmaceutical companies that make Aleve, Advil, Arthritis Foundation pain relievers, Tylenol and other analgesics are spending millions of dollars a year in the anti-arthritis race. And now who do we see coming from behind?

Aspirin!

Aspirin fell out of favor years ago, but a study published in the *Archives of Internal Medicine* suggests that it may be time to give aspirin another look. Researchers at Stanford University School of Medicine studied 3,000 people with rheumatoid arthritis and concluded that aspirin reduced pain and was relatively nontoxic.

Coated aspirin was found to be even less toxic.

Because aspirin is safe and much less expensive than any of the other nonsteroidal anti-inflammatory drugs (NSAIDs), the Stanford team suggests that aspirin may be an effective part of arthritis therapy after all.

That's good news for you and your pocketbook!

74. Donate One Pint of Blood

Every day, lives are saved because you or someone like you made blood available to someone who needed it. Tomorrow, your spouse, children or parents—or even you—may need donated blood to survive.

If you are in good health, weigh at least 110 pounds and are between the ages of seventeen and seventy-five, you can donate blood. In fact, if you are qualified, you can give blood four or five times a year.

Blood donation is *safe* and the whole process takes only about thirty minutes. Call your local American Red Cross or hospital for details on how you can become a donor.

The life you save may be your own.

75. Stockpile Your Blood

If you need an operation, consider stockpiling your own blood in case a transfusion becomes necessary during surgery. Research indicates that you have less risk of infection and other complications if you use your own blood rather than someone else's.

In a recent issue of *Lancet*, researchers reported that colorectal cancer patients who used their own blood had shorter hospital stays than those who used blood-bank blood. The researchers suggested that having blood drawn before surgery might boost immunity and even help prevent recurrence of the cancer.

76. Drink Up

Is your workplace hot—at least in terms of temperature? If it is, you should drink lots of water, especially if you're a man.

A recent study in the *Journal of Urology* reported that men who were exposed to high temperatures every day at an Italian glass factory's blast furnace had a higher frequency of kidney stones than co-workers in the same factory who worked in cooler areas.

The researchers concluded that dehydration caused higher levels of uric acid in the "hot" men—in fact, their uric acid levels were four times higher than those of their cooler co-workers—and the high levels of uric acid caused the stones.

The best way to prevent heat-induced kidney stones is to drink at least eight to ten eight-ounce glasses of water a day.

77. Pig Out on Greens

Make sure you have plenty of folic acid in your diet, particularly if you plan to get pregnant.

Folic acid plays a crucial role in the repair of cells damaged by everything from cigarette smoke to insecticide. It also helps your body produce red blood cells and reduces your risk of heart attack. Recent evidence also indicates that when pregnant women take folic acid, the nutrient can prevent neural tube birth defects.

Good sources of folic acid include asparagus, lima beans and dark green leafy vegetables.

The federal government's Daily Value (DV) for this essential vitamin is only 400 micrograms; you may need to take more if you're pregnant or planning to become so. Symptoms of a deficiency include anemia, diarrhea and a swollen, red tongue.

Talk to your doctor about how supplementing your diet with folic acid can help keep you in tip-top health.

78. Look Good for Fun and Profit

Take time every morning to make sure that you look your best. Researchers across the country have discovered that how you look can affect your inner chemistry. When you feel good about yourself, your body produces more of its own natural "feel good" chemicals—endorphins—which make you feel confident and relaxed.

Other researchers have found that paying attention to how you look can pay off in cash as well. According to researchers at Michigan State University, people who look good earn more money than those who do not. This advantage includes not only models and actors but also factory workers, construction workers and telemarketers.

79. Check Your Watch

Radium has been replaced by tritium in glow-in-the-dark watches in the past decade. But if you wear a watch with a plastic case, you may still be getting a dose of radiation.

A team of Australian researchers reported recently in the medical journal *Lancet* that a person who wears a glow-in-the-dark tritium watch with a plastic cover for three years receives about the same amount of radiation as people who lived in the Northern Hemisphere did from nuclear tests done in the 1960s. The researchers found *ten times* the amount of tritium in the urine of plastic-watch wearers as in the urine of people who wore conventional watches or no watches at all.

Next time you check your wristwatch for the time, check the kind you have. It may be time for a change.

80. Make Sure Your Cholesterol Test Is Accurate

Despite all the current hoopla over cholesterol levels, the blood tests given to check your cholesterol levels leave a lot to be desired. Some problems are caused by the equipment used. The tabletop machines used in public screenings can give varying results, from 200 to 250 for the same sample. But even the most sophisticated equipment can be off by 5 percent.

What can you do? Two things.

1. Always get a second test and compare levels.
2. Fast for twelve hours before a test to measure your HDL and LDL components.

Talk to your doctor about how often you should get your cholesterol checked.

81. Put Treatment Choices on the Record

If you or someone you know has had a heart attack, the good news is that aspirin can be a lifesaver. The bad news is that only 72 percent of people admitted to the hospital for heart attacks receive it.

In an article in the *Archives of Internal Medicine*, Charles Hennekens, M.D., and his colleagues asked why heart specialists seem to prefer extremely expensive drugs, such as streptokinase and tPA (which 25 percent of patients can't take), when aspirin can be given to almost anyone who doesn't have a family history of hemorrhagic stroke.

Ask your doctor what she or he thinks. Then have your doctor record those thoughts in your records at your local hospital. If you already have a Medic Alert bracelet or necklace, the information can be put on the record inside.

82. Weigh All the Factors

Since the 1960s, thin has been in. Models on TV, in magazines and on billboards seem to be thinner than ever.

Yet people over the age of forty can weigh ten pounds more than they did in their twenties and still be in good shape. In fact, because fat contributes to higher estrogen levels, a woman who weighs a bit more may experience fewer menopausal symptoms and have a lower risk of developing osteoporosis than if she weighed less.

Although the media glamorizes thinness, you may be better off carrying a few extra pounds. Ask your doctor to help you figure out your optimum weight.

83. Put a Stop to Violence

If there is violence in your home—whether directed at you or your children—you can stop it by leaving home or calling 911 if there is immediate danger. Or if the problem is just beginning, call your local domestic violence hotline—the number should be in the Yellow Pages under "Social Service Organizations"—and ask to speak to a counselor. You can do so without revealing your name.

Or reach out to a minister, priest, rabbi, therapist, family member or friend.

The important thing is to let someone know you need help today. You don't have to go it alone.

84. Wash Away Acne

Contrary to popular opinion, you don't get acne from eating oily foods. You get it from increased amounts of male sex hormones called androgens. These hormones, which naturally increase during puberty in men and during pregnancy in women, stimulate the production of sebum, an oily substance that can become trapped in the hair follicles on the skin. If too much sebum is produced, acne can result. Men have more and worse acne than women because they have more androgens.

The best thing you can do is gently wash your skin with an antibacterial soap twice a day. Never pick or squeeze pimples. Don't use a rough brush on your face. Antiseptic creams and lotions that contain benzoyl peroxide can help dry up pimples.

85. Talk to a Friend about Drinking

Sometimes silence kills as much as alcohol. If you have a friend who drinks too much, talk to him or her about it—the risks are too great to ignore.

Alcoholism is a progressive disease for which there is no cure, experts agree. The only successful treatment is abstinence. And many drinkers become abstinent by joining local chapters of Alcoholics Anonymous, seeking counseling or entering detoxification programs in hospitals.

Unfortunately, denial is an essential part of alcoholism. By talking to your friend, you may put the first crack in the wall of denial.

To learn more about alcoholism, call Alcoholics Anonymous, Al-Anon, the National Council on Alcoholism, your local health department, a local hospital, your union or the employee assistance program where you work.

86. Be Wary of Over-the-Counter Medications for Psoriasis

Many over-the-counter medications on the market that claim to treat psoriasis promise a lot but deliver little—and they can delay proper treatment.

Psoriasis, which takes the form of red, scaly patches covered by silvery white scales, affects about seven of every 100 Americans. Doctors don't know the cause but do know that it seems to run in families and that recurrences may be connected to emotional stress or to the physical stress of an illness such as strep or an upper respiratory infection.

Ultraviolet sunlamps—used according to your doctor's directions—can help, as can prescription-strength lotions and lubricants such as topical steroids. Special baths and shampoos, such as Neutrogena's T/Gel, also help remove scales.

87. Tense Your Muscles to Relax

Progressive muscle relaxation (PMR), developed in the 1930s by Edmund Jacobson, is a great way to release tension. With PMR, you work with four muscle groups.

Group 1   Forearms and biceps
Group 2   Feet, calves, thighs and buttocks
Group 3   Chest, stomach and lower back
Group 4   Shoulders, neck, throat, face and head

To see how effective PMR can be, sit in a comfortable chair or lie down on a comfortable bed or sofa. Breathe deeply and slowly. Then when you feel relaxed, tense the first muscle group. Hold the muscles tense for about ten seconds. You may feel a slight burning sensation. Let the muscles go limp and relax. Repeat this procedure twice. Work on the first muscle group for two or three days, then move to the second muscle group, the third and finally the fourth.

Experiment with PMR and find out what works best for you. Go slowly. Don't tense any muscle group so much that it hurts.

88. Count on TENS to Relieve Pain

If you have chronic pain, you may want to purchase a small device known as a transcutaneous electrical nerve stimulation (TENS) box.

TENS produces mild electrical pulses through electrodes that are taped to your skin. With TENS, you have control over where, when and how long you can find pain relief. The impulses from the TENS box send signals right to the nerves. These signals overload your pain circuits and block pain messages. TENS produces a vibrating, tapping or tingling sensation. It doesn't hurt.

Researchers have found evidence that, in addition to overriding pain signals in your body, TENS stimulates the release of endorphins—the body's natural painkillers—in the brain and spinal cord.

You control the intensity of the TENS signal by turning a dial on the box. Some people achieve long-term pain relief after using TENS for a short period of time. Others need TENS on a daily basis.

89. Avoid Headache-Causing Snacks

Those frequent headaches you get may not be caused by your boss, your spouse or the kids. It may simply be what you're eating.

Just as there are foods that stimulate pleasure, there are some foods that cause pain, especially headache pain. Common culprits are foods that contain the amino acid tyramine: alcohol, aged cheeses, inner organ meats such as liver, yeast extracts, sour cream, yogurt, vinegar and relishes, salad dressings, ketchup and chocolate. Foods with nitrites, nitrates or caffeine can also cause headaches.

If you think food is contributing to your headaches, try eliminating the above foods—one at a time—from your diet. If the pain goes away when a particular food does, you have probably identified the food that is causing it. Consult with a nutritionist to help you develop a pain-free eating plan. If headaches persist, consult a doctor.

90. Ask a Hypnotist for Help

Hypnotic "trances" were a part of medical practice in ancient Greece. In Europe in the 1800s, Franz Mesmer revived interest in the role of hypnotism in healing. And at the turn of the century, Sigmund Freud used hypnosis to explore the human mind.

Today, research into the healing applications of hypnosis is being carried out nationwide. There is renewed interest in hypnosis among physicians, psychiatrists, psychologists, social workers and other health professionals.

Hypnotism is not a miracle cure, but it can provide help for many health problems, including chronic pain. It can also help fight anxiety, depression, and addictions such as smoking and help to rebuild low self-esteem and restore lost confidence.

Ask your doctor to recommend an experienced hypnotist if you feel this technique may be of help to you.

91. Hypnotize Yourself

Train yourself to enter a trance, and achieve great benefits from self-hypnosis.

In the beginning, you can use a commercially made "induction" tape—available at most tape and record stores—to get into the trance state. If you are already working with a trained hypnotist, you can make your own tape.

First, become as relaxed as possible. Focus all your attention on your breathing and relax your muscles. Then imagine that you are descending deeper and deeper into comfortable darkness. Slowly count backward from ten to one to deepen the trance. Imagine a special place where you can be safe and peaceful. At this point, powerful hypnotic suggestions can be made that can reduce pain, promote feelings of vitality and energy, and enhance confidence and self-esteem.

To come out of your self-induced trance, begin counting from one to ten. Sit quietly for a few minutes to be certain you are completely out of the trance state.

Most people find the trance experience soothing and enjoyable. Other benefits, such as pain relief, are wonderful extras.

92. Massage Away Foot Pain

You can get quick, effective relief from foot pain by following these four steps:

1. Sit barefoot in a comfortable chair, drape a towel over your lap, then put your right foot on your left thigh. Rub your foot gently, using a massage oil or lotion. Use both thumbs to apply pressure to the sole of your foot.

2. Make a fist and move your knuckles up and down the sole of your foot. Do this five times.
3. Massage each toe individually. Hold the toe firmly between your thumb and index finger and move it from side to side.
4. Hold your foot steady with your left hand. With your right hand, take hold of all your toes and bend them backward, holding them in that position for five to ten seconds. Do this three times.

Repeat this procedure with your left foot. With regular massage, your feet will feel so good that they won't mind walking the 100,000 miles most of us will walk in a lifetime!

93. Try Acupuncture

Acupuncture has been practiced for almost 5,000 years and is available in more than 100 countries today. It is becoming increasingly popular in the United States, and experienced acupuncturists are opening practices in cities, suburbs and even rural areas.

Many conditions respond to acupuncture treatment—asthma, allergies, colds, sinusitis and chronic pain, to name but a few. It is safe and effective and has few, if any, side effects.

In acupuncture, thin needles are inserted at precise points on the body. The needles block pain signals. Researchers have found that acupuncture also improves circulation, relieves muscle tension and stimulates the production of endorphins, the body's own natural painkillers.

If you have a medical problem that is not responding to traditional medicine, talk to your doctor about giving acupuncture a try. The results may surprise you.

94. Say Good-Bye to Pain

If you are sick and tired of living with chronic pain, it's time for you to find a nearby pain clinic, so you can get some R-E-L-I-E-F!

There are more than 1,000 pain clinics in the United States today. Ask your doctor to recommend one near you. A good pain clinic will offer a complete line of services, including all of the following:

Trigger point injections
Nerve blocks
Transcutaneous electrical nerve stimulation (TENS)
Acupuncture
Biofeedback
Total relaxation training
Self-hypnosis training
Guided imagery training
Physical therapy
Movement therapy
Individualized exercise programs
Assertiveness training
Behavior modification
Group therapy

If medication or self-help techniques are not helping to reduce chronic pain, it may be time to make an appointment with the experts at a nearby pain clinic.

95. Try Biofeedback

Learn to change and control your response to stress with biofeedback. Biofeedback isn't a form of therapy. It's a way for you to monitor your response to stress by giving you objective information about your heart rate, muscle tension, skin temperature and blood pressure—all of which indicate how tense or relaxed you are.

A biofeedback specialist puts electrodes and sensors on your body, and a biofeedback monitor shows whether you're relaxed. If you are experiencing stress, the specialist will help you learn how to relax.

Most people need about twelve biofeedback sessions with a specialist (once or twice a week, one hour at a time).

The specialist probably will also provide you with an instructional audiotape you can follow to continue biofeedback at home. You can learn to take your own pulse, to use a mirror to see your muscles relax and to measure your own body temperature with an inexpensive "ring thermometer." For more information, call the Association for Applied Psychophysiology and Biofeedback in Wheat Ridge, Colorado, at 303-422-8436.

96. Pat Yourself on the Back

How you think about yourself determines what you do in life. If you think something is impossible, it is. If you think something is possible, you may make the effort needed to achieve it.

Research in the field of cognitive therapy has proven that you can change the way you think, and when you change how you think, you change how you behave.

To help you see yourself as someone who makes things happen, make a start at changing your thinking. Get a pen and paper, and in one column, write down any criticisms you have of yourself. In a second column, write down all your positive characteristics, talents and attributes.

Which column was easier to fill up? For many people, it's the negative one. And just realizing that, then struggling to find more "positives," can make a big difference in how you live each day and in how much you enjoy life.

97. Make a Three-Pronged Attack against Extra Weight

On New Year's Eve, did you make a resolution to get a handle on your "love handles" this year? A recent survey in the *New York Times* revealed that seven out of ten New Year's resolutions had to do with health—and most of them involved weight. Yet few areas of health are as inundated with fads and quackery as the area of weight. And few are as obviously and immediately connected with self-esteem and self-worth.

It's important to be as close to your ideal weight as possible because excess weight puts a strain on your heart, lower back, hips and knees. Some research even suggests that being overweight may put you at risk for developing osteoarthritis.

Talk to your doctor today about developing a gradual, balanced program of exercise, nutrition and stress reduction that will help you keep your commitment to yourself and lose those unhealthy extra pounds.

98. Be Your Own Massage Therapist

You can lower stress and sometimes reduce pain by giving yourself a massage.

How massage exerts its soothing effects is not completely understood. But blood flow increases to the part of your body being massaged, and the physical stroking, kneading and rubbing relax the area.

Massage is most effective for relieving muscle stiffness and spasm, but research also indicates that it sends pleasure signals to the brain. In fact, these electronic bursts of pleasure can frequently overcome pain signals being sent from the same area.

Some people find that powders or oils help their hands glide more smoothly over the skin, increasing the effectiveness of the massage.

Talk to your doctor about the role self-massage can play in increasing your energy and vitality as well as in reducing stress in your life. There are also many excellent books available on massage, such as *The Book of Massage* by Lucy Lidell, *The Massage Book* by George Downing and *Massage for Common Ailments* by Sara Thomas.

99. Watch What You Eat before You Exercise

Most people feel invigorated after exercise, but a few develop allergic reactions: They break out in hives, develop itching palms and soles or experience wheezing and other breathing disorders.

According to an allergist at Harvard Medical School and Brigham and Women's Hospital in Boston, exercise alone does not cause an allergic reaction. What does is eating foods such as apples, peaches, cabbage, celery and shellfish before you start to sweat.

To avoid this problem, the researchers recommend that you wait for four hours after eating before you begin to exercise. And if you are exercising and feel any allergy symptoms, stop exercising and consult a doctor. If you're having difficulty breathing, call an ambulance.

100. Choose a Health Club Near Home or Work

How many people do you know who join a health club in a burst of enthusiasm and then almost never go? Membership in a health club can provide many benefits—but only if you use it.

Common sense dictates that you can increase the chances that you'll go to your health club regularly if you choose one that's within fifteen minutes of work or home.

The club's schedule should match yours as well. Is it open before work, after the kids have gone off to school or on weekends? Is it open at night?

There are many other important factors to consider when

choosing a health club, such as cost and adequate staffing, but convenience to home or work is at the top of the list.

101. Be Good to Your Back When You Touch Your Toes

Even the simplest exercise can be hazardous if you don't do it right. To avoid injury, be careful about which exercises you choose to do and how you do them.

Toe-touching the old-fashioned straight-legged way keeps the knees locked in place and puts tremendous pressure on the lower back, which can result in significant pain. And that plus rapid movements up and down can also cause injury.

If you want to do toe-touching exercises, bend your knees slightly, lean over and touch your toes, staying in a "hanging-over" position for three complete, deep breaths. Perform this activity—without bouncing—three times. Then slowly straighten.

102. Sit Up Right

Sit-ups are a great way to build a strong abdomen, but doing them improperly can cause serious problems.

Don't do sit-ups with your legs out straight. This will increase the curvature of your lower back. Try doing your sit-ups this way: Lie flat on your back, with your knees bent and your feet flat on the floor. Fold your arms across your chest. Now curl your shoulders up from the floor at about a thirty-degree angle, then lower them back to the floor. This will give your abdominal muscles all the exercise they need without putting you in danger of injuring your lower back.

If you're not sure how to do an exercise correctly, don't do it at all until you talk to an expert at your local YMCA, fitness club or community center.

103. Make the Medicine–Exercise Connection

Sometimes two things that are good for you on their own can be dangerous together.

If you take aspirin before you begin exercising, for example, the drug may prevent you from feeling pain that's signaling your body to stop exercising. And as a result, you may continue to exercise and injure yourself.

Other medications can raise your blood pressure or cause drowsiness when combined with exercise. To be safe, always ask your doctor how any new drug you're taking works with exercise.

104. Never Mix Aspirin and Vitamin C

During the cold and flu season, you get lots of advice on how to fight the symptoms that come with these illnesses. Many people swear by vitamin C for both prevention and treatment, and most people will take an aspirin or two at some point during a bout with any illness.

But both vitamin C and aspirin are acids. Vitamin C is ascorbic acid, and aspirin is salicylic acid. And if you take these two substances at the same time, they can irritate your stomach. Researchers have found that heavy doses—which people often take to fight cold and flu symptoms—can produce severe stomach irritation that may lead to the development of ulcers.

105. Relieve Pain with Acupressure

Relief for your headache may be at your fingertips—literally. You can use acupressure, a form of acupuncture, for fast relief.

A part of Chinese medicine for thousands of years, acupressure works on nerves that are just below the skin surface at special points throughout your body. Although no one knows why acupressure works, the results speak for themselves.

Try this technique for yourself. To relieve your headache, apply very heavy—almost painful—thumbnail pressure just above the bone that protrudes on the thumb side of your wrist. Or apply pressure to the triangle of skin between your thumb and your index finger on the back of your hand. Remember, you need to apply heavy pressure.

After you practice acupressure a few times, you may find that relief is just an acupressure-point away.

106. Use Lavender to Lull You to Sleep

If you're going through a period when it's hard to fall asleep, try a little lavender oil in your bath. Researchers in England recently reported that lavender oil has a light sedative effect. It not only helps people fall asleep, it also helps improve the quality of sleep.

Although researchers have plans for more formal studies using people of all ages, you may want to conduct your own personal "experiment" by sprinkling a few drops of lavender in your bath. You'll be continuing a 1,000-year-old tradition, since even the ancient Romans used lavender as a folk remedy.

107. Ask Your Surgeon Tough Questions

Surgery is always serious and risky. Ask for the information you need before you decide to have an operation.

Among the questions you should ask the surgeon are:
1. What risks do I face?
2. What is the mortality rate for this procedure?
3. How many of these operations have you done in the past year? What is your mortality rate?
4. What kinds of post-op drugs will you prescribe, and what are their potential side effects?
5. How long until I'll be back to normal?
6. What kinds of complications can occur, and how frequent are they?

7. Do some of your patients choose not to have this procedure even though you recommend it? Why?
8. What other options are available?
9. Can you recommend a physician for a second opinion?

We now describe doctors as "health care providers" and patients as "consumers." Medicine is more of a business now than ever. Protect yourself by asking questions.

You can get additional information from organizations such as Ralph Nader's group, Public Citizen, 2000 P Street NW, Suite 605, Washington, D.C., 20036 (202-588-1000).

108. Learn Hospital Lingo

Have you ever been in the hospital when a doctor or nurse came in to discuss your ills—and you couldn't understand half of their words? Every profession has its own "jargon," and medicine is no exception. Here are some common medical terms and their definitions.

Iatrogenic: doctor-caused
Nosocomial: hospital-caused
NPO: patient receives no food or drink
hs: medication before sleep
IV: intravenous
BP: blood pressure
Medication schedule: qud—four times daily; tid—three times daily; bid—two times daily; od or qd—once daily; qod—every other day
PRN: as needed

Whenever you, a family member or a loved one is in a hospital and you don't understand what a member of the medical staff has told you, ask her to explain it in a way that makes sense to you. It's her job.

109. Use a Good Toothbrush and Use It Well

A toothbrush may seem like a pretty easy purchase to make, but take some time to make sure that your toothbrush is right for you.

Generally, a soft nylon toothbrush works best. Nylon brushes dry out more quickly than brushes with natural bristles, and soft bristles are less likely to damage your gums than firmer ones.

Also, buy two toothbrushes and use them in rotation. This will allow each brush to thoroughly dry. If you get a cold, you may want to buy a new toothbrush when your cold is over. Germs can continue to live in the brush, and you can reinfect yourself.

A recent study revealed that the average person spends thirty seconds brushing his or her teeth instead of the recommended three to four minutes (although the people in the study estimated that they took more time brushing). Observe your dental hygiene habits, and if you have any questions, talk to your dentist.

110. Soothe Your Pain with Music

Got an ache in your hip? A pain in your knee? Instead of reaching for your usual over-the-counter pain reliever, try sitting back and listening to twenty minutes of music.

Why?

Music affects the cerebral cortex (the thinking part of the brain), the limbic system (the emotional part of the brain) and the brain stem (the primitive part of the brain). And some researchers have even found evidence that music stimulates the body to produce *endorphins*, the body's own natural painkillers.

At Kaiser Permanente in Los Angeles, doctors use music to help patients with disorders that can be aggravated by stress, such as high blood pressure, ulcers, back pain and migraines. Physicians also use music in combination with biofeedback and hypnosis to relieve chronic pain.

Would you rather put on a tape or a CD of soothing music than take an aspirin? Try it. You may find that the soothing sounds of your favorite performers are just what the doctor ordered.

111. Talk to Your Doctor about Treatment for Osteoporosis

If you are one of twenty million American women with some form of osteoporosis, talk to your doctor about a new treatment that may soon be available. A slow-release form of fluoride and calcium nitrate has been shown to increase bone density and reduce the number of bone fractures by up to 83 percent in some patients.

Osteoporosis is a disease in which the bones thin and become brittle. The results can become crippling over time as fractures occur in the spine, hips and wrists. In particular, microscopic spinal fractures can cause back and leg pain and a curvature of the spine called dowager's hump.

Yet the new treatment seems to create solid bone. Although more studies are being undertaken, even skeptics in the medical field seem convinced that a breakthrough is at hand.

112. Get the Root That Gets to the Root of Insomnia

If you have bouts of insomnia even though you're getting exercise, managing stress and avoiding alcohol and caffeine, you may be interested in an herbal approach.

Recent scientific studies have shown that valerian root, a widely used folk medicine, has sedative properties that can improve the quality of your sleep and relieve insomnia. Studies show that, unlike many prescription and over-the-counter sleeping pills, valerian has no "hangover" side effects.

Scientists compared valerian with other drugs in subjects who took them under laboratory conditions and found valerian to be as effective as mild doses of benzodiazepines (tranquilizers such as Valium).

If you decide to try valerian, take it thirty to forty-five minutes before you go to bed. It's available as a dried root tincture or extract. Follow package instructions, but if you find that you're sleepy in the morning, reduce the amount you're taking. You can purchase valerian at most health food stores. For more information, call the Herb Research Foundation in Boulder, Colorado, at 303-449-2265.

113. Pay Attention to Your Prostate

Among men ages twenty to forty, inflammation of the prostate caused by bacteria or a virus is the most common health problem. Symptoms include a frequent, urgent need to urinate, sexual difficulties such as premature ejaculation and impotence, and discomfort in the lower abdomen and genital area. In these circumstances, you need to see a doctor.

114. Make Love after a Heart Attack

Not only is it safe to have sex after a heart attack, but the pleasurable activity of making love is good for you, too! Just ask your doctor when you're recovered enough to give it a go—and whether or not you should take any medication to prevent chest pain during your activities.

There are a few things you can do to make the experience less physically stressful. Foreplay not only is fun but also helps the heart gradually get ready for increased activity. And it's probably best to engage in sex when you are most relaxed—in the morning or perhaps after an afternoon nap.

The period of recovery from a heart attack can be a difficult time. But the pleasure, intimacy and emotional closeness that come from making love with your partner can help speed the healing process and bring peace of mind.

115. Adopt a Fertile Lifestyle

Infertility is a problem that is on the rise in the United States, and male infertility has been given more attention in recent years. If this is a concern of yours, consider making a few minor—but important—lifestyle changes before you rush off to see an expensive specialist.

The main problems in male infertility are sperm count, the mobility of the sperm produced and the quality of the sperm. Alcohol, caffeine, cigarettes and "recreational drugs" affect sperm count and mobility and lower testosterone levels. Using any of them can prevent you from becoming a parent.

You may find it difficult to quit smoking, cut out coffee and stop drinking, but by doing so, you may find the easy answer to infertility.

116. Ignite Your Sex Life

Researchers have discovered evidence suggesting that regular exercise may make you sexier!

New studies indicate that exercise stimulates production of hormones such as testosterone in both men and women. And this increased production of sexual hormones may cause an actual chemical increase in libido.

What's more, exercise makes you look and feel sexier, too. It helps you lose weight and keep it off. It boosts your self-esteem and helps you fight anxiety and depression.

Overall, exercise makes you feel and look "mah-velous," as Billy Crystal used to say.

(Where did you put the schedule for that exercise class?)

117. Make Sure Medication Isn't Lowering Your Libido

Illness can reduce your desire for sex, but some widely prescribed drugs can also pull the plug on your sex life.

If your libido seems low and you're taking tranquilizers, antidepressants or medication for high blood pressure or digestive problems, ask your doctor if your medication could be zapping your sex life. You may be able to take a lower dose of the drug you're taking, or you may be able to switch to a different one that doesn't reduce your libido.

118. Outwit Montezuma

Everyone has heard the warning "Don't drink the water" when traveling to different countries around the world. But if you slip and drink the water or forget that ice cubes are no-no's, a common over-the-counter medication may save your vacation.

Researchers at the University of Texas performed an experiment with 128 students who visited Mexico. The students were divided into two groups. One group was given bismuth subsalicylate (the active ingredient in products such as Pepto-Bismol); the other group was given placebos.

Only 22 percent of the students given bismuth subsalicylate developed diarrhea. The group given the placebos did not do as well; 60 percent of them developed diarrhea while abroad.

You may want to consider taking bismuth subsalicylate as the students in the experiment did—four tablespoons four times a day for twenty-one days—to help prevent this extremely common traveler's health problem.

119. Imagine Your Cold Away

Recent research in the area of visualization suggests that the pictures you create in your mind may actually be able to help fight off a cold because they help strengthen your body's immune system—quickly, safely and effectively.

How do you do it?

It's simple. When you get up in the morning, relax by taking slow breaths that get deeper and deeper. Focus all your attention on your breathing. Then imagine descending into the center of your body. Visualize yourself in a safe, peaceful place where you're bathed in a warm, soft, golden light. Then imagine that your body's own healing cells are flooding the parts of your body affected by the cold and fighting off the illness. See yourself feeling strong, without any of your cold symptoms. Every few hours during the day, take five minutes to relax and visualize yourself getting better. In the evening, spend another fifteen minutes visualizing.

Visualization may seem an unusual way to fight a cold, but give it a chance. It just might work!

120. Select a Nursing Home Carefully

Selecting a nursing home can be a painful process. But once you've decided that you or a family member needs one, you can help ensure that the choice you make is the healthiest one for you and your family.

First, contact the American Health Care Association (202-842-4444) and the American Association of Homes and Services for the Aging (202-783-2242), both in Washington, D.C., for tips on selecting a nursing home. Then contact your state agency on aging or a church or community organization to get listings of local nursing homes. Make sure that the homes are accredited, licensed and certified for Medicaid and Medicare.

Then make your first visit to the nursing home without an

appointment. Perform your own "sniff test" to make sure the home does not smell of urine. Check to see that it is clean, safe and uncrowded. Listen to hear if any staff are yelling at residents. Visit the dining area at mealtime and inspect the kitchen. Talk to residents to see how they like living there. Find out what kind of regularly scheduled activities the nursing home offers its residents and sit in on some sessions. Note how many staff members are around and whether they're primarily trained nurses or unskilled orderlies.

Other important factors to consider include attractiveness of surroundings, ongoing staff training and cost.

121. Love Away Back Pain

Studies indicate that sexual activity can relieve pain for hours or days at a time, and it can be a pleasurable way to soothe a sore back. Positions least likely to cause additional strain on your back include the following:

- Front-to-back: The man lies behind the woman so that the two are nestled together like spoons.
- Face-to-face: The partner with the back pain—man or woman—should lie back-down, perhaps using a pillow under the knees for increased comfort. His or her partner stays on top.

These are not the only ways a couple can continue to make love when one partner has a bad back. Experiment and see how many other positions you can add to your repertoire.

122. Measure Your Stress

Did you ever notice that some people seem to roll along easily through life while others seem to be tripped up at every turn? It is your reaction to events, not the events themselves, that causes the kind of stress that leads to a vulnerability to serious health problems such as heart attack and cancer.

One stress expert has devised a simple stress test you can use to evaluate your level of stress.

Imagine that you are in the supermarket in the express lane. You can only have up to ten items in your cart in this lane, but the person in front of you has twelve.

On a scale of one to ten, rate your level of stress over this incident. How much does it bother you? Now on a scale of one to ten, rate how important this event is in your life. The difference between those numbers is a good indication of your stress level. If you rated the incident in the supermarket a six in bothering you but only one in importance, for example, your stress level would be a five—high in comparison to the event's importance.

How can you reduce the level of your reaction to various events? Actually, just being aware that you tend to get stressed out fairly easily is enough to begin modifying your reaction.

123. Prime Your Pump

Every day, your heart pumps more than 2,000 gallons of blood through 60,000 miles of blood vessels in your body. With every heartbeat, 300 *trillion* cells receive nourishment.

That's a lot of work. But your heart will keep working for a long time if you're good to it. And a good diet is one important way to keep it healthy.

The American Heart Association has established some easy-to-follow dietary guidelines to help you reduce your risk of heart disease:

1. Eat a wide variety of foods, so your body will have a broad base of nutrients from which to meet its needs.
2. Limit your alcohol consumption.
3. Don't overeat.
4. Keep your total fat intake under 30 percent of your total daily calories.
5. Keep saturated and polyunsaturated fats under 10 percent of total daily calories.

6. Get 50 percent of your daily calories from complex carbohydrates such as pasta and potatoes.
7. Keep cholesterol under 300 milligrams a day.

124. Put More Emphasis on Protein

You may want to consider rearranging your diet to conform with the numbers 40-30-30—which means 40 percent protein, 30 percent carbohydrates and 30 percent fat.

While there is continuing debate over what combination of protein, carbohydrates and fat is good for you, many people are adopting this particular formula. And they say they feel trimmer, more energetic and healthier overall since changing their diets.

The 40-30-30 system was developed at Stanford University in the late 1980s and has been popularized in a book by Barry Sears called *The Zone*. The basic theory of the diet is that if you eat too many carbohydrates—such as bread, pasta and potatoes—it will be difficult for your body to burn excess fat.

There are no exact studies to definitively prove that the 40-30-30 diet is the last word on the subject. But if you haven't found quite the right diet for yourself, the 40-30-30 may be worth a try.

125. Shine a New Light on Your Cholesterol Problem

If you have high cholesterol levels, the answer for you may be spelled L-I-G-H-T.

Diet, exercise and drug therapy are the mainstays in the struggle to lower cholesterol levels and to keep those levels down. But research performed at the University of Texas Health Science Center has shed new light on the cholesterol problem. The researchers have found that cholesterol levels can average 6.4 points higher in the winter than in the summer. As a result, at least one biologist predicts that light may be effective in treating unhealthy cholesterol levels.

Ask your doctor if he or she thinks that natural sunlight—or full-spectrum lightbulbs in the home—may help you reduce your cholesterol levels.

126. Reduce Your Risk of Heart Disease

Heart disease is the number one killer of both men and women in the United States. But you can reduce your risk of developing it by making a health plan for yourself that includes:

- Stopping smoking
- Avoiding alcoholic beverages
- Exercising regularly
- Maintaining a desirable weight
- Having your blood pressure and cholesterol levels checked regularly
- Eating a balanced diet (low in total fat, saturated fat and dietary cholesterol; high in fruits, vegetables, whole grains and fiber)

Take the time to look at your lifestyle and see how you can adopt these sensible health suggestions.

127. Try a Little Tenderizer

Scientists say the best remedy for a bee sting may be found in your kitchen, not your medicine cabinet—meat tenderizer!

According to a researcher at Stanford University, the toxins in the bee's stinger that cause the pain are actually forms of protein. The research performed at Stanford indicates that these proteins can be broken down by using meat tenderizer. Mix regular meat tenderizer with water, then apply it to the painful area, researchers suggest. This should reduce your discomfort.

If you're allergic to bee stings, or if you experience any swelling, however, head for the nearest emergency room.

128. Educate Yourself on Mammography Equipment

There is disagreement among doctors over when a woman should have a mammogram. Some recommend a "baseline" mammogram at age thirty-five, followed by yearly mammography beginning at age forty. Other doctors think that women don't need mammography until age fifty. At times, even large organizations such as the American Cancer Society and the National Cancer Institute don't recommend the same course of action for doctors and patients.

One thing that everyone agrees on, however, is that it's critical that the equipment be of the best quality available.

The American College of Radiology (ACR) certifies mammography facilities based on its own stringent standards. You can call the ACR at 703-648-8900 to see if the facility you are going to is ACR-certified. Ask for the mammography department when you call.

129. Ditch Deodorants and Talc before You Have a Mammogram

To get the best "pictures" possible, don't use a deodorant or talcum powder on the day of your mammogram.

The talc in the powder and the aluminum hydroxide in the deodorant are absorbed through the skin in the underarm area. These materials can then pass into breast tissue and possibly show up on the mammogram as calcium deposits.

Calcium deposits in breast tissue are one of the signs indicating that cancer is present. So by using talcum powder or a deodorant before your test, you could create the conditions that would result in a false-positive test result. In other words, your mammogram would indicate cancer where there is none.

Don't worry about perspiration on the day of your exam. You can take care of that after you have had your mammogram.

130. Add Years to Your Life at Lunchtime

Take a brisk walk for thirty minutes or so every day at lunchtime and add years to your life.

How?

A brisk walk burns almost as many calories as jogging. Plus, it raises your metabolism, tones your muscles and lifts your mood. The result is a healthier life.

A recent study by the Cooper Institute for Aerobics Research showed, for example, that moderate everyday activity such as walking provides significant protection from cardiovascular disease, cancer and a host of other disorders. The study was carried out over an eight-year period and involved more than 13,000 men and women.

So get away from your desk at lunchtime and take a walk. You'll be doing something good for your health, and you'll likely be more energized all afternoon!

131. Don't Try to Be a "Super Mom"

A mother who works has two jobs: The first one begins when she gets everyone else off to work and school, and the second one starts when she arrives at her own job. When she gets home, her first job picks right up again.

If you're a working mother, you're probably working twice as hard as your husband, even if he helps out around the house. And if you're working and raising your children alone, you have an even more difficult burden. Here are a few tips to keep both you and your kids happy, healthy and sane.

- Set aside some time to do something just for yourself.
- Delegate some responsibility for household chores to your kids.
- Schedule your tasks and stick to your schedule.
- Reward yourself every now and then for all the work that you do.

132. Stay Calm and Live Longer

Do you explode every time the slightest thing goes wrong? Do you have a cynical attitude toward people?

If you answered yes to either of these questions, you may have to change your way of thinking and behaving if you want to live a long and satisfying life.

Angry, cynical people are five times as likely to die before age fifty as people who are calm and trusting, according to studies undertaken by a psychiatrist at the Duke University Medical Center. The studies indicate that acting out anger toward others and a cynical mistrust of people are strong predictors of premature death.

If you nearly burst a blood vessel when a shoelace breaks or believe that no good deed goes unpunished, you may want to give some thought to changing your attitudes. They may be more damaging to your health than you think.

133. Use Your Head—And Protect It

Bicycling is a wonderful, healthy activity, but use your head when riding your bike.

More and more people are taking up bicycling as part of a healthy lifestyle, but an old habit may prove dangerous or even fatal. As a kid, you probably rode a bike without a helmet. Yet five out of six deaths from bicycle accidents are caused by injuries to the head and neck—and all the evidence indicates that helmets would have prevented those injuries.

Always wear a helmet when you ride your bike—and set an example for your children to follow.

When buying a helmet, look for the American Natural Standards Institute (ANSI) or Snell Memorial Foundation (SNELL) seal of approval.

134. Choose Sunglasses with UV Coating

Look for the "UV100" tag on any pair of sunglasses you buy. It's your guarantee that your eyes are protected from the premature aging caused by ultraviolet rays.

Fewer than half of the sunglasses on the market have adequate protection from ultraviolet light, so you have to be careful.

Many people think that dark glasses provide protection—and the darker, the better. But dark lenses without UV coating may be more dangerous to your eyes than wearing no sunglasses at all. Dark glasses cause your pupils to dilate. And with your pupils opened more widely, you're likely to receive an even larger dose of ultraviolet radiation than if you weren't wearing sunglasses at all.

135. Avoid Blue Sunglasses

Color counts for more than looks in sunglasses. You may want to choose blue shades because they match your eyes, but they can be dangerous.

According to an eye specialist at the Manhattan Eye, Ear and Throat Hospital in New York City, you are better off with lenses that are tinted yellow or amber. These lenses are more protective of your eyes because they transmit yellow light, which is less damaging than the blue light transmitted by blue lenses.

Good lenses don't need to be expensive, either. For as little as eight dollars, you can get sunglasses that will provide effective protection against damaging rays.

136. Let Your Shadow Show You the Way

Your shadow will tell you when it's safe to go out in the sun and when it's better to stay in the shade.

When your shadow is shorter than you are, the sun's rays are at their most intense. Usually, this will occur from 10 A.M. until

2 P.M. (or from 11 A.M. until 3 P.M. in daylight saving time), just when the sun's radiation is most dangerous.

If you cannot avoid being out at that time—or if you want to be in the sun at the beach or poolside—be sure to wear a hat to protect your head and plenty of sunscreen to protect exposed areas of your body.

Your sunscreen should have a sun protection factor (SPF) of at least 15. Apply the sunscreen generously and reapply it every two hours. Then you can enjoy the sun without fear of premature aging or cancer.

137. Call a Chiropractor

If nothing seems to be working for your pain and your family physician can't seem to help, make an appointment for a consultation with a chiropractor.

Thousands of years ago, Hippocrates (the father of Western medicine) said, "In case of illness, look to the spine first." Although the American Medical Association (AMA) fought chiropractic for decades, today many "regular" doctors refer patients to chiropractors for help.

Chiropractic was founded in 1895 by David Daniel Palmer and is based on the belief that the relationship between the spine and the nervous system is central to health and well-being.

Doctors of chiropractic are licensed practitioners who provide conservative management of, and help prevent, neuromusculoskeletal disorders and related functional clinical conditions, including, but not limited to, back pain, neck pain and headaches. They are expert providers of spinal and other therapeutic manipulation/adjustments.

Contact the American Chiropractic Association at 1-800-986-4636 for the name of a doctor of chiropractic near you.

138. Patient, Heal Thyself

Take responsibility for your own health.

According to one of the top health experts in the country, David E. Bresler, Ph.D., who works at the Los Angeles Healing Arts Center, the key to creating a healthier you is to intensify your motivation to live a healthy life.

How?

You can begin to take responsibility for your health by taking an honest look at how you are living. How can you change your life to make yourself happier and healthier?

For instance, maybe now is the time to quit smoking. Or maybe you want to get serious about cutting alcohol from your life. Whatever you decide to change to improve your health, make it your priority to succeed. Give it all you've got.

You have the power to create a new, healthier you today.

139. Pray or Meditate

Maybe science isn't really opposite to faith, after all. New research in medical science supports the ancient belief that there is a role for prayer and meditation in healing.

Studies indicate, for example, that seriously ill people are more likely to get well if they're prayed for than if they're not—even if they don't know that anyone is praying for them!

In fact, prayer is apparently such a powerful tool that Larry Dossey, M.D., author of *The Power of Prayer*, even incorporates prayer into treatment plans for his patients—as do a surprising number of doctors in America.

No matter what your religious affiliation, or whether you are religious at all, you may find the act of praying comforting and relaxing, and it may even be a good way to relieve chronic pain. A wide range of books and materials is available to get you started. *The Seven Spiritual Laws of Success* by Deepak Chopra may be helpful for the nonreligious, while *Care of the Soul: A Guide for Cultivating Depth and Sacredness in Everyday Life* by Thomas Moore may be helpful for people of traditional faiths. Pick up either of these books at your local bookstore or library and explore the possibility of prayer or meditation in your life.

140. Manipulate Stress Away

The Feldenkrais method, a movement technique developed by physicist Moshe Feldenkrais, has been used by actors, dancers, professional athletes and people with special problems such as cerebral palsy to eliminate stress and tension in their bodies.

The instructors who teach the technique use gentle muscle manipulation to show students how to move more naturally. The Feldenkrais method includes a group approach and private individual sessions. The instructors are not doctors.

The technique can help reduce pain from a muscle injury, and even chronic pain, by reducing muscle tension. You may find that when your tense muscles relax, you feel less emotional and mental stress as well.

To learn more about this technique, read *Awareness through Movement* by Dr. Feldenkrais or attend a workshop in this technique. They are given all across the country. For more information, call the Feldenkrais Guild in Albany, Oregon, at 503-926-0981.

141. Move in New Directions

The Alexander Technique is a method designed to help eliminate negative movement patterns that can cause muscle aches and strains. It was developed by the actor Frederick Alexander as he attempted to solve certain problems he faced onstage.

The Alexander Technique helps you develop a greater awareness of your everyday physical habits—how you walk, sit and stand. Most of us have developed poor ways of doing these things, so you are taught new, more natural ways to move through the world.

You may find that as your old ways of moving are replaced by new ones, you no longer have chronic problems that once troubled you, such as lower back pain, sciatica, muscle aches and headaches.

You can learn more about this technique by reading *The Alexander Technique* by Wilfred Barlow or *The Alexander Technique* by Edward Maisel. You can also take classes to learn the technique. For more information, call the North American Society of the Teachers of the Alexander Technique at 1-800-473-0620.

142. Learn to Pace Yourself

Modern life is moving faster and faster, but that doesn't mean you can't apply a little "stopping power."

How?

Take a quiet break during the day. A few minutes of rest is important on the job, at home and even when on vacation. People who are always on the go may soon burn out and be gone!

A quiet moment of meditation in the office will make you more productive during the workday. A peaceful period will help a homemaker stand up to the stress of managing a household and caring for children and a spouse. And a few minutes of quiet will prevent a vacation that is crammed with activities from becoming physically and emotionally draining instead of rejuvenating.

143. Affirm Yourself

Create a positive statement about yourself and use it to fight negative feelings that arise during the day.

Experts in cognitive therapy, such as Martin E. Seligman, Ph.D., author of *Learned Optimism*, have proved that what and how you think influences your health—and that you can change the way you think to improve your health.

One way is to develop and use positive statements. To give it a try, get into a relaxed state of mind. Create a simple affirmation, such as "I am a loving person." Always state your affirmation in the present tense and make it positive. Then feel the positive sensations that course through you as you make your affirmation.

Bookstores are filled with hundreds of books containing affirmations. One of the best ones is Shakti Gawain's *Reflections in the Light—Daily Thoughts and Meditations*.

144. Go All Out for the "Deep Heat"

Try some of the available deep-heating lotions the next time you have a massage.

Massage is a soothing, comforting experience that is enhanced by the addition of oils and lotions. And although deep-heating lotions do not directly relieve aches and pains, as most advertising would have you believe, some of these rubs contain medicines that block pain sensations, while others increase blood flow to the skin where they're applied—an effect that speeds healing.

If you don't know a good massage therapist, ask your doctor for a recommendation.

145. Let Someone Touch You

What you might need most right now is to be touched.

Practitioners say that touch—called therapeutic touch when it's intended to heal—produces healing and reduces pain through a transfer of energy from one person to another. And although scientists aren't sure what it means, research suggests that hemoglobin levels are higher in the blood of subjects treated with therapeutic touch than in those not treated by this technique.

It may be that therapeutic touch transfers a healing power that can help all of us: love.

146. Use a Security Blanket

We all need comfort sometime during the day, and a "solacing object" may bring you the security you need.

For a child, a "security blanket" may be a blanket, baseball glove or doll. For an adult, it may be a photograph of a spouse or children or a paperweight that sits on the desk as a reminder of a good friend.

All of these are examples of what are called solacing objects. And although they may seem sentimental, they are eminently practical because they can evoke powerful memories of happy times with loving family members and close friends. The emotions that are stirred by the memories can help relieve pain, reduce anxiety, fight depression and sometimes bring feelings of peacefulness and safety.

At times in this chaotic world, we each need to feel safe. Keep something with you that will bring you comfort when you most need it.

147. Make a Personal Health Plan

Making a personal health plan that outlines what you do to stay healthy can help you take control of your health.

Use a blank book, a spiral-bound book, a ring binder or any other convenient format to record your plan. The following are some of the items you may want to keep track of:

- Medications: what you take and when to take it
- Exercise schedule: what exercises you engage in and when
- Relaxation exercise schedule: what relaxation techniques you use and when
- Healthy habits you're working on, such as eating more vegetables and walking
- Questions for your doctor
- Important phone numbers: your doctor, pharmacist, therapist and other health care providers and any health organizations that are important to you

A written health plan can prove invaluable because it keeps you on track and thinking about your health.

148. Know What Drugs to Take

Each year, Americans spend close to $100 billion to relieve acute or chronic pain with non-narcotic and narcotic drugs. Non-narcotic drugs are not addictive. They include aspirin, acetaminophen, ibuprofen and sodium naproxen. All are effective at relieving mild to moderate pain and sometimes even severe pain.

Narcotic drugs, which are used to relieve short-term severe pain, can be addictive. Although most people don't get hooked on narcotic medications, the potential is always there. That's why you should take these powerful drugs cautiously.

If you have any doubts about their impact on you, speak to your doctor candidly. There may be effective alternatives.

149. Make Your Favorite Chair a Healthy Chair

You can prevent or minimize back pain by ensuring that you always sit in a chair that gives your back the support it needs.

Whether you are at home or at work, the best kind of chair to use is a firm recliner that has contoured support and an adjustable lower back cushion.

If you do a lot of sitting in your car—commuting to and from work or shuttling the kids or aging parents around the neighborhood—check out the design of your seat. You need a seat that gives support to the curve of your spine.

In general, Japanese and Swedish cars have better-designed seats. But the best way to find what suits you is to pay attention to seat design when you are test-driving a car.

150. Be Informed

Information is power, and it is crucial in today's changing health care landscape.

You may no longer have a relationship with a personal physician, and you may have had to change health plans a few times as well. So where can you get health information that you can rely on?

The organizations below provide reliable medical information. Some charge a fee, others don't.

- Center for Medical Consumers Library in New York City, 212-674-7105
- The Planetree Health Resource Center at the Institute for Health and Healing in San Francisco, 415-923-3680
- Health Resources in Conway, Arkansas, 501-329-5272 (fee)
- Medical Information Service in Menlo Park, California, 1-800-999-1999; or the Medical Information Service in Palo Alto, California, 415-853-6000 (fee)
- National Health Information Center, a federally funded referral service; call 1-800-336-4797 to reach a number of organizations

151. Put Pepper on Your Pain

In the 1600s, Montezuma put hot chili peppers in his hot chocolate. In the 1800s, Irish doctors used them for tooth pain. And today, American doctors use capsaicin—the active painkilling ingredient in peppers—to relieve pain from rheumatoid arthritis, osteoarthritis and shingles.

Researchers think that capsaicin blocks pain by depleting one of the chemicals your body needs to send pain signals to the brain. In one study of 100 patients with arthritis who used Zostrix, a drug that contains capsaicin, 57 percent of the participants experienced reduced pain. They were able to perform daily tasks more easily, and some were even able to exercise regularly after using capsaicin.

A number of over-the-counter products contain capsaicin as

the active ingredient. Ask your doctor or your pharmacist to help you choose one.

152. Take a Bath before Bed

To ensure a good night's sleep, treat yourself to a hot bath about two hours before bedtime.

Sleep researchers have found that a hot bath—at least 103 degrees Fahrenheit—raises your body temperature so that when you later crawl under the covers, your temperature begins to fall. As it does, report the researchers, it sets off strong sleep signals, so you drift into a deeper sleep.

153. Position Yourself to Prevent Pain

You can prevent a great deal of back pain by learning muscle-friendly ways to bend, reach and lift.

If you have to lift or move heavy objects—get help!

Then remember to keep your back flat and straight when picking something up. Pinch your buttocks together, tighten your stomach muscles and rotate your pelvis forward. And avoid twisting when lifting by putting your feet forward, facing the object, before lifting. Don't lift objects higher than your shoulders or hold them lower than your knees.

If you have to reach overhead for an object, use a ladder, a footstool or a long-handled tool. Avoid straining a muscle by reaching overhead yourself.

154. Use a 12-Step Program to Reduce Pain

Follow the 12 steps below, and you will have control over any chronic pain in your life.

The director of the Pain Treatment Center at the Scripps Clinic and Research Foundation in La Jolla, California, has devised this comprehensive, easy-to-follow pain control program which uses the 12-step model pioneered by Alcoholics Anonymous.

1. Accept your pain.
2. Distract yourself from pain with recreation, hobbies or work.
3. Get angry at your pain.
4. Take all medications as prescribed.
5. Use relaxation techniques.
6. Get fit and stay fit.
7. Keep active.
8. Pace yourself.
9. Ask for help from family and friends.
10. Be open and honest with your doctor.
11. Share your experiences with others who have chronic pain.
12. Stay hopeful.

155. Pop Pills Properly

Make sure you take any painkillers properly, so you get the maximum effect.

Popping pills to fight pain may seem an easy thing to do, but there are some important tips you should follow when using these drugs, whether they are prescription or over-the-counter.

First, always use the weakest painkiller you can to fight pain. Second, take the analgesic on a fixed schedule. This makes it easier to control the pain. Third, take the recommended dosage, so you maintain a constant level of the drug in your blood system. And fourth, use your medication to "stay ahead" of your pain and keep it controlled. In this way, you can avoid the need for higher dosages or stronger drugs.

156. Use Eyebrow Massage to Relieve Headaches

Give yourself an eyebrow massage to get fast pain relief for tension headaches, migraines or sinus headaches.

It's a simple technique that's easy to learn and even easier to do. Just run your index finger along your eyebrow. You will notice that at one point there's a "dip." This is the spot you're looking for—right near the center of your eyebrow. It's at this point, doctors say, that the supraorbital nerve comes close to the skin's surface.

Sit down and press on this point on both eyebrows, using the knuckles of your thumbs. Keep pressing until you feel pain. If you don't feel any pain, you are not applying pressure to the correct spots. Shift your thumbs a fraction and try again.

Apply this pressure for about fifteen to thirty seconds. Your headache should go away in minutes.

157. Try Nontraditional Medicine for a Bad Back

If your back is bothering you, you may not want to see a doctor.

A recent survey of people with back pain produced some surprising results. According to the survey, of the 492 people questioned, only 23 percent of those who saw orthopedists for back pain experienced moderate to dramatic long-term pain relief. And only 4 percent of patients who saw neurologists experienced significant pain relief.

Yet chiropractors helped 28 percent of their patients, and acupuncturists brought relief to 36 percent of theirs.

Even better, yoga instructors helped 96 percent of patients, dance instructors helped 90 percent and psychiatrists helped 86 percent.

So who is most likely to help you with back pain? If you have chronic back pain that your doctor can't fix, you may want to consult someone with a different approach than traditional medicine.

158. Make a Relaxation Tape

Make an audiotape to help you relax. Three elements must be included on the tape: breathing, suggestive phrases and progressive muscle relaxation.

To get started, place a tape recorder on a table beside you, turn the volume up to 80 percent of maximum and press the record button. Then sit in a comfortable chair and let your body relax. Pay attention to your level of stress as you begin, but focus your attention on your breathing. Breathe in deeply, all the way to your diaphragm, then slowly exhale.

Breathe deeply for several minutes, and then when you feel relaxed, repeat a suggestive phrase such as "My feet feel warm and heavy" until your feet feel warm and heavy. Tighten and then relax the muscles in your feet as you speak. Repeat this procedure with all the muscle groups in your body, working progressively from your feet to your head and back to your feet. Any tension you feel will drain away. Play the tape every day, and follow your own voice to that laid-back feeling.

For more information on how to make a relaxation tape, look in your library or bookstore. There are many excellent books available on this topic.

159. Add Vitamins to Your Life

A varied diet usually provides adequate amounts of vitamins, minerals and other nutrients. But sometimes it can't satisfy all your nutritional needs—such as when you're ill, pregnant or taking medication.

Talk to your doctor. He or she may suggest that you take a good multivitamin or larger amounts of a few specific vitamins.

All vitamins come with the Daily Values on their labels. The Daily Value represents the amount you need to prevent a deficiency in that vitamin (and it may actually be much lower than the amount you need to take).

160. Go All the Way with Vitamin A

Vitamin A is needed for good vision; for healthy tooth, bone, skin and hair development; and for strengthening cell walls, so they can fight infection.

The Daily Value of vitamin A is 5,000 international units (IUs). But you may need to take more, especially if you have any deficiency symptoms such as night blindness or rough, scaly skin.

You can get vitamin A from milk. Dark green vegetables and deep yellow fruits such as peaches and cantaloupe are good sources of beta-carotene, which turns into vitamin A in your body. Carrots, sweet potatoes, pumpkin and squash are also excellent sources of beta-carotene. Natural sources are generally preferred over supplements, since supplements of vitamin A can be toxic, especially when taken by pregnant women.

Talk to your doctor about how this essential vitamin can keep you healthy and full of energy.

161. Take Time for Thiamin

You may want to add thiamin—also known as vitamin B_1—to your diet. Vitamin B_1 is essential for healthy heart and nervous system functioning and is needed to help your body break down carbohydrates into energy. This vitamin also plays an important role in regulating your appetite, in growth and in maintaining proper muscle tone.

Good sources of thiamin are pork and other lean meats, oysters, green peas, collard greens, asparagus, beans or legumes, whole grains and oranges.

The Daily Value for thiamin is 1.5 milligrams. But you may need to take more than that amount, especially if you are experiencing any of the common deficiency symptoms, such as leg cramps, muscle weakness, loss of appetite, confusion, forgetfulness, or moodiness or irritability.

Ask your doctor about how supplementation with this essential vitamin can fit into a diet that will keep you healthy and energetic. Any B vitamin supplement should be taken only under a doctor's supervision, since too much can cause nerve damage—and even just a little of one B vitamin can cause deficiencies in others.

162. Eat Riboflavin-Rich Foods

Vitamin B_2—or riboflavin—is an essential nutrient that helps your cells effectively use oxygen. It also plays a key role in helping your body turn protein, carbohydrates and fat into new cells.

You can get riboflavin from lean meats, chicken, oysters, sardines, tuna, dark green vegetables, legumes and whole grains.

The Daily Value for vitamin B_2 is 1.7 milligrams. But you may need to take more than that amount, especially if you are experiencing any deficiency symptoms such as cracks at the corners of your mouth, a rash around your lips or nose, or hypersensitivity to light.

163. Be Nice to Yourself—Take Niacin

Niacin—or vitamin B_3—is essential for your cells to effectively use oxygen and to properly metabolize protein, carbohydrates and fat. It also promotes healthy skin and a hearty appetite.

You can get niacin from lean meats, poultry, fish, dark green vegetables, legumes, nuts and whole grains.

The Daily Value for niacin is twenty milligrams. But you may need to get more than that amount, especially if you're experiencing any deficiency symptoms such as skin rashes, indigestion, diarrhea, irritability, depression, anxiety, confusion or a red, swollen tongue.

Talk to your doctor about how supplementation with this essential vitamin can fit into a diet that will keep you healthy and energetic. But remember, don't take one B vitamin without the others. Otherwise, you could cause a deficiency in one of the ones you're not taking.

164. Get Plenty of B$_6$

Vitamin B$_6$—or pyridoxine—needs to be a part of your diet.

This essential vitamin plays an important role in helping your body form red blood cells and in maintaining a balance between sodium and potassium. Vitamin B$_6$ is also needed for your body to metabolize protein, carbohydrates and fat effectively.

You can get vitamin B$_6$ from lean meats, poultry, fish, corn, legumes, nuts, whole grains and bananas.

The Daily Value for vitamin B$_6$ is two milligrams. But you may need to take more than that amount, especially if you're experiencing any deficiency symptoms such as cracks at the corners of your mouth, a rash, anemia, depression, irritability or dizziness.

Talk to your doctor about how your diet can be supplemented with this essential vitamin to help keep you healthy and energetic. Remember, however, that supplementing one B vitamin can cause a deficiency in the others.

165. Improve Your Overall Health with Vitamin B$_{12}$

Add foods rich in vitamin B$_{12}$—or cyanocobalamin—to maintain normal growth and to replace spent red blood cells, which carry oxygen and nutrients throughout your body. Vitamin B$_{12}$ is involved in maintaining the balance between sodium and potassium in your body. It also keeps your nervous system healthy and helps your body metabolize protein, carbohydrates and fat.

You can get vitamin B$_{12}$ from lean meats, fish, shellfish, dairy products and egg yolks.

The Daily Value for vitamin B$_{12}$ is only six micrograms, but you may need more than this amount, especially if you experience anemia, tingling or numbness in your fingers, or fatigue.

166. Take Breaks from Your Computer

Take regular breaks when working at a video display terminal to avoid the eyestrain and muscle pain and stiffness that are common among people who use their computers a great deal.

Every two hours or so, go for a walk around the block or to a different part of your workplace.

To prevent stiffness and pain in your neck, frequently stretch your shoulders and lower back. Some exercises—such as shrugging your shoulders or rotating your head clockwise, then counter-clockwise—can be performed in your chair. Others—for example, bending at the waist—should be done while standing. And blink your eyes frequently to help keep them moist.

167. Know How to Handle Nosebleeds

You can stop a minor but frightening problem—and maybe prevent more serious trouble—by learning how to stop nosebleeds more effectively.

A few simple steps can handle most cases of nosebleed, according to the American Academy of Otolaryngology. First, sit with your head leaning forward. Using your thumb and index finger, pinch your nostrils closed. Keep a gentle pressure on your nostrils for about fifteen minutes and breathe through your mouth. Next, apply a cold compress to the nose area and keep it there while you are holding your nose closed.

After the bleeding stops, don't blow your nose for at least twenty-four hours. Try not to bend over so that your head is lower than your heart.

If the bleeding doesn't stop, or if it starts up again shortly afterward, call your doctor. The nosebleed may be a symptom of a more serious problem.

168. Fight Bad Breath the Easy Way

If you have bad breath, it can usually be eliminated through good oral hygiene.

First, brush your teeth more frequently and don't forget to floss, so you can reach the places your toothbrush misses. Bad breath is usually caused by decaying food particles that remain in the mouth after meals.

After you've brushed and flossed, brush your tongue, as it can become coated with bacteria that produce an unpleasant odor. You may also want to pick a mouthwash and use it as directed.

These simple actions—plus regular visits to your dentist for cleanings—should clear up most cases of bad breath. If the problem persists, see your dentist. You may have gum disease—or even a stomach or lung problem.

169. Soothe a Sore Throat

Gargle with ordinary water and salt, suck on a lozenge or have a warm drink to ease sore throat pain.

Sore throats are usually caused by viruses or bacteria. See your doctor if the pain is severe or if you have a high fever and other serious symptoms. Otherwise, every two to three hours, mix one-half teaspoon of salt into a small glass of warm water (four to six ounces) and gargle with the solution. Frequently sip tea with honey or other warm beverages.

Sucking on a medicated lozenge or even a piece of hard candy can also be very soothing.

170. Learn How to Take Your Temperature

Your body temperature fluctuates throughout the day. But if your temperature is over ninety-nine degrees Fahrenheit (as measured by an oral thermometer), it's safe to assume you have a fever.

Overlooking simple things can cause inaccurate readings. If you use an oral thermometer shortly after drinking a hot liquid, for example, you may get a high reading when you don't have a fever at all. You may also get a false reading if you take your temperature too soon after exercising. And women's temperatures can be affected by hormonal changes in their bodies, such as those that occur around ovulation.

To make sure you get an accurate reading, sit down and avoid eating or drinking anything for at least fifteen minutes before you take your temperature.

171. Add Pantothenic Acid to Your Vitamin Arsenal

Your body needs pantothenic acid to metabolize protein, carbohydrates and fat. It also plays an important role in your body's ability to make hormones and other chemicals that regulate the nervous system. Fortunately, pantothenic acid is found in fresh vegetables, whole grains and egg yolks.

The Daily Value for this vitamin is only ten milligrams, but you may need to take more than that amount if you are experiencing any deficiency symptoms such as severe abdominal cramps, nausea, fatigue, tingling in your hands or feet, or sleep problems.

Talk to your doctor about supplementing your diet with pantothenic acid.

172. Buy Into Biotin

Your body uses biotin to release energy from the protein that you eat. It helps break down carbohydrates and fat and plays a role in the formation of fatty acids. Biotin works in conjunction with the other B vitamins that are a part of your healthy diet.

You can get biotin from dark green vegetables, green beans, cauliflower, legumes, mushrooms, nuts and egg yolks.

The Daily Value for biotin is only 300 micrograms, but you may need to take more if you're deficient. Although biotin deficiency is rare, it does occur. Eating raw egg whites can result in the destruction of your body's biotin, while certain metabolic problems can also interfere with biotin.

Talk to your doctor about boosting your body with biotin.

173. See What C Can Do for You

Vitamin C prevents the destruction of B vitamins, helps your body absorb iron and enables your body to fight infections. It also helps wounds heal and assists your body in making collagen, which holds the cells together. It may also reduce cholesterol and help prevent cancer.

You can get vitamin C from oranges and other citrus fruits and their juices. Other good sources include cantaloupe, strawberries, brussels sprouts, broccoli, green peppers, collard greens, asparagus, cauliflower and tomatoes.

The Daily Value for vitamin C is only sixty milligrams, but you will probably need more, as sixty milligrams is only the minimum needed to prevent scurvy.

You may need higher doses of vitamin C if you have swollen, red or bleeding gums; swollen, aching joints; nosebleeds; or a wound or an infection that is slow to heal.

Talk to your doctor about supplementing your diet with C.

174. You Deserve Your D Today

Children who don't get the proper amount of vitamin D may experience poor bone growth. Overall growth can also be impaired, and muscles and teeth will not be as strong as they could be. Adults who don't get enough vitamin D can suffer softening and weakening of the bones and loss of bone calcium.

Vitamin D helps your body absorb and metabolize calcium and

phosphorus. It plays an important role in the development of healthy teeth and bones. There is even some evidence that this vitamin may protect some people against colon cancer.

Sunlight helps in the formation of vitamin D. You can get this vitamin from fortified milk, fortified cereals and egg yolks.

The Daily Value for vitamin D is 400 international units (IUs), but you may need to take more. Talk to your doctor about adding more D to your diet.

175. Make Things Okay with Vitamin K

Vitamin K is produced by bacteria that live in your intestines. Babies do not have these bacteria at birth and are often given vitamin K in the hospital. The vitamin activates enzymes that are needed to stimulate your body to produce the chemicals that promote blood clotting. It also triggers the manufacture of proteins that prevent the clotting from spreading to other parts of your body. Vitamin K helps your body regulate calcium in the blood as well.

You can get vitamin K from green leafy vegetables, milk, egg yolks and liver.

There is no Daily Value for vitamin K, but research indicates that it is safe at levels of 70–140 micrograms. It's almost impossible, doctors say, to have a deficiency, since the body can make its own vitamin K. Nevertheless, if you have delayed blood clotting or if you bruise or hemorrhage easily, talk to your doctor about whether or not you should increase your consumption of vitamin K–rich foods.

176. Make Minerals a Meaningful Part of Your Life

Although there is debate among doctors and researchers about whether diet alone can supply all the minerals you need or whether mineral supplements are required to maintain health, there is no disagreement over the fact that nutrients such as calcium and iron are critical to good health and vitality.

Your body requires significant amounts of the "major" minerals (such as calcium, magnesium, phosphorus, potassium, sodium and sulfur) and smaller amounts of the "trace" minerals (such as chromium, copper, fluoride, iodine, iron, manganese, molybdenum, selenium and zinc).

What's the best way to make these minerals part of your life?

Eat a varied diet that emphasizes fresh fruits and vegetables, whole-grain breads and cereals, plus low-fat dairy products such as yogurt and milk.

177. Get Calcium-Rich Today

Calcium is necessary throughout life for strong bones and teeth and for normal heart functioning. Calcium also plays a major role in blood clotting and is vital to the healthy operation of your nervous system. For adults, the most serious consequence of not getting enough dietary calcium is osteoporosis, a condition in which your bones become brittle and break easily. Children who don't get enough calcium will have stunted growth.

Low-fat milk and other dairy products are excellent sources of calcium. You can also get calcium from sardines and salmon (eaten with the bones), green leafy vegetables, tofu, oysters, clams, and citrus fruits.

The Daily Value for calcium is 1,000 milligrams, but you may need to eat more calcium-rich foods if you have a family history of osteoporosis.

178. Unleash Magnesium's Magic

Magnesium helps your body build protein, release energy from the foods you eat and relax muscles after they contract. In addition, it's necessary in fighting tooth decay and in transmitting nerve impulses throughout your body.

Good sources of magnesium are wheat germ, bran and other whole grains as well as dark green vegetables, legumes, nuts and seafood. You may be surprised—and happy—to learn that chocolate and cocoa are good sources as well!

The Daily Value for this mineral is 400 milligrams. You may need to eat more magnesium-rich foods, however, if you are experiencing deficiency symptoms such as muscle weakness, nervousness, confusion or disorientation. Deficiencies of magnesium are not very common, but they do occur when other medical problems are present.

179. Use Phosphorus to Get the Most out of Food

Your body needs phosphorus to activate the nutrients that you get from foods and supplements. Phosphorus helps make teeth and bones strong and plays an important role in helping your body get energy from food. It also helps in sending impulses along your nervous system.

Milk and dairy products are good sources of phosphorus, as are lean meats, poultry, fish, legumes, nuts, whole grains and egg yolks. You can also get phosphorus from some processed foods and soft drinks.

The Daily Value for phosphorus is 1,000 milligrams. You may need to eat more phosphorus-rich foods if you are experiencing deficiency symptoms such as muscle weakness or bone pain.

Deficiencies of this mineral are not common, but they can occur when other medical problems are present.

180. Put Potassium to Work for You

Potassium is needed for your heart to function properly and for your body to maintain fluids and acids in balance. In addition, your body uses this mineral for muscle contraction, for the transmission of signals along your nervous system and for storing energy.

You can get potassium from lean meats, fresh vegetables, fresh fruits, milk and other dairy products, nuts, and legumes. Many salt substitutes also contain potassium.

The Daily Value for potassium is 3,500 milligrams. A potassium deficiency can sometimes result in muscle weakness, irregular heartbeat and other physical symptoms. A potassium deficiency usually occurs only if you experience excessive loss of fluids, through diarrhea or heavy sweating, for example. If you are using diuretics, you may become deficient in potassium.

Talk to your doctor about how much of this essential mineral you need to stay healthy and energetic.

181. Drink Eight Glasses of Water a Day

Make a habit of drinking at least eight eight-ounce glasses of water every day.

Two-thirds of our planet and two-thirds of your body are composed of water. It is probably the most essential of all the essential nutrients, although most adults in the United States do not consume enough.

Your body needs water for proper digestion, to keep mucous membranes moist, to dispose of bodily wastes and to perspire, a process that keeps your body cool. Water is also essential for a healthy bloodstream.

182. Keep Your Hands Clear of Viruses

Reduce your risk of catching a cold by being careful about what and whom you touch.

Recent studies have shown that the common cold—which will affect about thirty million Americans this year—isn't transmitted by coughing and sneezing alone.

Colds are spread primarily by hand. If someone with a cold gets the virus on his or her hands, you can catch the cold by shaking that person's hand, drying your hands with a towel that person has used or by picking up money handled by that person. You can then spread the cold virus in the same ways.

Minimize your risk of getting a cold by washing your hands frequently and avoiding touching other people and their belongings unnecessarily. Use disposable tissues when you blow your nose, cough or sneeze instead of covering your mouth and nose with your hand.

The odds are that you will be one of the three in four people in the United States who get colds this year, but you can cut those odds significantly by watching what and whom you touch.

183. Learn What Pulls the Asthma Trigger

Asthma affects about ten million Americans. It's a physical illness, although an internal chemical cascade triggered by strong emotion can also cause an attack.

In an asthma attack, muscle spasms in the lungs' air passages cause the airways to narrow. The result is the wheezing, coughing and breathing difficulties associated with an asthma attack.

Asthma attacks are frequently brought on by breathing pollen, animal dander, mold particles, dust or smoke. Certain foods can bring on an episode for some people, and drugs—prescription and over-the-counter—contain ingredients to which some people are allergic. Even exercise has been known to cause an asthmatic episode.

Keep a record of asthma attacks and the circumstances surrounding them. You may be able to identify asthma triggers and eliminate them from your life.

184. Control Allergy Attacks

You can control allergic attacks of sneezing and sniffling by learning what allergens trigger an attack.

Keep a record of your attacks, noting when and where they occurred and what you were doing at the time. If you start coughing and sneezing and your eyes water when you're in the yard, don't mow the lawn or rake the leaves yourself. That will reduce your exposure to pollen from grass, trees and weeds—not to mention the molds—that may be causing your problem.

You may find that you start having an allergic response in your bedroom. Keep the bedroom free of dust, molds and other allergens. You may want to cover pillows and mattresses with plastic covers or install an air conditioner or air purifier for the room.

Whatever the season, by dusting and vacuuming frequently, washing area rugs and getting rid of objects that collect dust, you can live more comfortably.

185. Cool Your Burning Heart

Many competing drug companies are flooding the airwaves with commercials for new heartburn products, a number of which are weaker versions of the drugs used to treat ulcers. But before you resort to these over-the-counter cures for heartburn, try avoiding heartburn in the first place.

The heart is not involved in heartburn. The pain you feel is caused by stomach acid that slips up into the esophagus from your stomach and causes pain.

Among the common triggers for heartburn are alcohol, coffee, garlic, onions, peppermint, aspirin, heavy meals and eating too quickly. Smoking after a meal can also bring on heartburn.

Try eliminating these triggers one by one to see which one—or ones—is causing your heartburn. If heartburn persists, see your doctor to rule out physiological causes such as hiatal hernia.

186. Keep Your Bowels on the Move

Constipation is a problem that plagues millions of Americans at one time or another. Usually, it's easily treated by good eating habits.

Add fresh vegetables, fresh fruits and whole-grain products

such as bran cereal to your diet. They contain fiber, which absorbs water and makes stools soft and easy to pass. And remember to drink plenty of water when you're eating high-fiber foods. Not only does your body need plenty of liquid for the fiber to absorb, but not enough water with a high-fiber diet can cause the very problem you're trying to cure.

If your problem seems serious or lasts for more than a day, call your doctor for advice. Sometimes constipation can be caused by a medication or by an underlying medical problem.

187. Pay Attention to Your Body's Signals

Constipation can cause a great deal of discomfort. If you're eating a healthy diet—with lots of fresh fruits and vegetables and whole grains—but still experience constipation, it may be your behavior that's causing the problem.

Everyone's body has its own "time to go." Ignoring your body's signals and refusing to accommodate its needs will result in chronic constipation. Eventually, in fact, your body may no longer let you know when it's time to head for the bathroom.

The world is moving faster, business is more demanding, and time is money—but don't put off a trip to the bathroom when you need to go.

188. Create Your Own Spa

At a spa, you're pampered, soothed and renewed. The luxurious treatment you receive from the health spa staff can energize you, relieve stress and help maintain your good health.

But you can turn your bathroom into a spa by the addition of a few inexpensive items. Turn off the overhead light and use candles for a soothing glow. Purchase a variety of incense scents and burn one each time you bathe to add to the luxurious feeling of your spa. Purchase special soaps, herbs and oils for your baths.

None of these products need cost very much, yet they can help turn a simple bath into an energizing and revitalizing experience.

189. Bathe Away Stress

Before bedtime, add a few drops of chamomile oil to a warm bath to relax your body and relieve stress.

The oil has a fragrance similar to apples, and when used as a bath oil, it helps relax tense muscles and soothe dry, irritated or itchy skin. The oil also has gentle sedative effects and helps promote a peaceful feeling. Anger, anxiety and sadness may seem to flow away into the warm waters of your bath.

There are many books on herbs available today that can give you further information about how to use this wonderful plant to ease tension and relax.

190. Use Cypress to Help Overcome Grief

For thousands of years, cypress trees have been planted in burial grounds and cemeteries. Is it a surprise that aromatic oil from the cypress can comfort the suffering?

By adding cypress oil to your bath, you may achieve a sense of peace and solace and a reprieve from the emotions that are troubling you.

In addition to adding cypress oil to your bath, you can use this oil to enhance the soothing, invigorating feelings you get from a massage. It also acts as an astringent for oily skin and hair.

Try a touch of cypress oil. You may come to value it as highly as the ancient Chinese, Egyptians and Greeks did.

191. Free Yourself with Frankincense

More than 5,000 years ago, the ancient Egyptians and Hebrews used frankincense in religious ceremonies. Its spiritual effects were thought to be so powerful that it was one of the three gifts the Magi gave to the baby Jesus.

The oil has a comforting scent. It helps deepen and slow your breathing. Often it produces a feeling of calm that helps create an atmosphere in which prayer or meditation can naturally occur.

While it helps lift your spirits, frankincense also helps tone the skin, can sometimes smooth away wrinkles and is an excellent treatment for oily skin. And because of its gentle, soothing properties, many women the world over use frankincense oil as a massage aid for childbirth.

Try this favorite of the ancients in your home spa, and you may come to greatly appreciate its effects.

192. Add Sensuality to Your Bath

For thousands of years, the fragrance of jasmine has been considered one of the most potent aphrodisiacs in the world. By adding jasmine oil to your bath, you may experience strong sexual feelings, which you can also express creatively in art, work or activity.

Many people also find that jasmine calms the nerves and inspires a sense of optimism and confidence. Some people even say that jasmine helps them overcome feelings of deep melancholy.

Jasmine will be a welcome addition to the herbs, oils and fragrances you keep in your home spa.

193. Get to Know the Mysteries of Myrtle

Add myrtle oil to your bath for a soothing, sensual experience.

Myrtle has a long history of use for emotional rejuvenation and physical healing. It was a favorite of the ancient Greeks and still is widely used throughout the Mediterranean region. In Europe in the sixteenth century, myrtle was a popular skin lotion and was used as an astringent. It was called angel water.

This oil cleanses the skin and has a subtle effect on the nerves and senses. It is very effective with children and with the elderly because of its gentle properties.

When you use this oil in a bath, it will become an important and useful part of your home health spa.

194. Look at the World from a Rose-Scented Bathtub

Rose oil can be healing for you physically, emotionally and spiritually. Since antiquity, the rose has symbolized perfect love and beauty. The tombs of the pharaohs, the temples of the ancient Greeks and Roman Catholic shrines to the Virgin Mary were all adorned with roses.

The fragrance of the rose was first captured in the tenth century by the alchemist Avicenna. It can lift your mood and bring you a feeling of self-confidence and general well-being. It is also a natural moisturizer for all types of skin and a gentle antiseptic and astringent.

195. Use Rosemary for Remembrance

Students in ancient Greece and Rome wore garlands of rosemary around their heads to increase memory and the ability to concentrate. You may find that adding rosemary oil to your bath relaxes you and makes concentration easier.

This oil, distilled from the evergreen shrub, seems to help overcome mental fatigue. It is useful in treating both dry and oily skin as well as acne, eczema and other skin problems.

196. Stimulate Yourself with Sandalwood

This aromatic oil is derived from the sandalwood tree, a slender evergreen that is now endangered. In the East, sandalwood is used as an aphrodisiac, as a means of reaching a higher spiritual level and as a spur to creativity. Its soothing scent aids in meditation and brings joy to many people.

Sandalwood oil in the bath can bring you relief from stress and anxiety and sometimes can even help relieve mild depression. And it can help dry, chapped skin because of its natural moisturizing properties.

When used as a bath oil or as part of a massage, responsibly-harvested sandalwood oil can reduce your stress and leave you feeling rejuvenated.

197. Erase Stress from Your Face

Try your own blend of Eastern oils to nourish dry skin, refresh your spirit and erase the effects of stress.

Put ten drops of geranium oil and twelve drops of bergamot oil into an empty ten-milliliter bottle and top it off with camellia oil or sweet almond oil. Put the cap on firmly and tilt the bottle back and forth at a ninety-degree angle. Don't shake the bottle.

Pour a touch of the oil into the palm of one hand, dip the fingertips of your other hand into it and apply the oil liberally to your face and neck, avoiding your eye area. Gently massage your face and neck with your fingertips, using upward strokes.

To reduce tension, move your fingers slowly across your forehead, first left to right, then right to left. Using your index finger, gently massage the circumference of your mouth, moving your finger in clockwise circles.

Then sit quietly, breathing in and out. Enjoy the results of your beautiful, stress-reducing facial.

198. Learn the Warning Signs of Heart Attack

Heart attack is the leading cause of death in the United States, yet most people don't recognize its signs and wait too long to call for help.

Part of the problem is that not all heart attacks will happen in precisely the same way. According to the American Heart Association, however, the most common warning signs are:

- Uncomfortable pressure, feeling of fullness, squeezing or pain in the center of your chest that lasts two minutes or longer
- The spread of pain to your neck, shoulders or arms
- Dizziness, sweating, nausea, fainting, shortness of breath or severe pain

None of these symptoms is always present. A symptom may appear, subside, then return again.

If you think that you or someone else is having a heart attack, call an ambulance.

199. Lower Your Heart Attack Risk

Some heart attack risk factors are due to heredity, but a great many are under your control.

Get a piece of paper and a pen. Make three columns on the page. In the left column, under the heading "Risk Factors," write down the main heart attack risk factors: smoking, high blood pressure, overweight, high cholesterol, lack of exercise, high stress. In the center column, under the heading "My Health," rate your health by writing yes or no next to each category, according to whether or not it pertains to you. Then in the right column, under the heading "My Prevention Plan," write down how you intend to change your lifestyle so that you can reduce your risk of heart attack.

Putting your plan in writing can be the first important step to taking action.

200. Erase Pain

If you experience headaches, jaw pain, lower back pain, arthritis, bursitis, shinsplints, "tennis elbow" or another painful condition, myotherapy may be a great help to you.

Bonnie Prudden, a leading authority on physical fitness and exercise who helped to create the President's Council on Physical Fitness and Sports under President Eisenhower, believes that 95 percent of all pain starts in your muscles and that there are trigger points in muscles that cause pain when they are activated by physical or emotional stress. Her technique, called Pain Erasure, focuses its attention on these trigger points.

You can learn how to apply pressure to your muscles using your fingers, muscles and elbows to bring quick pain relief. Go to the library or bookstore and ask for the book *Pain Erasure, The Bonnie Prudden Way*. It will give you both the theory and the practical techniques of this excellent pain relief program.

201. Limit Your Exposure to X Rays

You may not think twice when a doctor or a dentist tells you that you need an X ray. But according to John Gofman, M.D., Ph.D., professor emeritus at the University of California, Berkeley, Americans receive too many.

When someone suggests you get an X ray, ask why you need it. Sometimes X rays are ordered for legal, not medical, reasons, and you may want to refuse them. If you are seeing a doctor for a second opinion, take the X rays from the first physician with you. If you change dentists or are going for an examination by a dental specialist, take your X rays with you.

X rays can be of great help, but they also have the potential to do harm. Always ask for X-ray shields or lead aprons for the parts of your body not being X-rayed.

202. Cut On-the-Job Risks

Learn the health and safety rules that apply in your workplace and follow them.

Wear any protective clothing and devices that are provided or recommended, including equipment to protect your ears from excessive noise, safety glasses to protect your eyes from injury and masks or other respiratory equipment to protect you from breathing hazardous fumes.

Exposure to hazardous substances can cause heart or lung damage or injure your skin, eyes or ears. Overexposure to a single industrial agent or to a combination of agents may cause cancer, according to the American Cancer Society. Certain agents—nickel, chromate, uranium, asbestos and petroleum vinyl chloride—are known to cause cancer.

203. Spice Up Your Health with Cinnamon

Cinnamon has been used since ancient times in Greek, Italian, Indian and Moroccan cooking. In the United States, this delectably aromatic spice is frequently used in baked goods, cereals and herbal teas.

But cinnamon has long been known also to have medicinal, as well as culinary, benefits. It increases circulation, reduces flatulence, helps control diarrhea and may even reduce pain from menstrual cramps.

In addition, cinnamon oil has shown evidence of antibacterial action. It can help fight staphylococcal germs and *Candida albicans*, or thrush.

And Max de Roche, author of *The Foods of Love*, claims that cinnamon even acts as an aphrodisiac.

Add the spice of cinnamon to your diet, and add to your health and joy in life.

204. Take Coated Aspirin

If you take coated aspirin, also called enteric-coated aspirin, you can avail yourself of aspirin's benefits and reduce the risk of its possible adverse side effects.

A recent study, reported at a meeting of the American College of Gastroenterology, found that people who used coated aspirin had less gastrointestinal bleeding than people who took regular aspirin. The researchers found that the advantages of coated aspirin existed even when low doses were taken.

According to the researcher who conducted the study, people who took plain aspirin had more than twice the amount of bleeding of subjects who took coated aspirin.

If you sometimes have trouble tolerating aspirin but wish to use it regularly to reduce pain or protect your heart, coated aspirin may be a good idea.

205. Create Your Own Health Library

You can put together a sophisticated health library of your own that's always available for reference.

National health organizations such as the American Cancer Society and the American Heart Association offer excellent free pamphlets and booklets on the prevention and treatment of disease. The numbers of the local chapters are in your phone book.

The United States government is another source of valuable health information. The various branches of the National Institutes of Health (301-496-4000) and the U.S. Department of Agriculture are among the divisions of the federal government in Washington, D.C., that you can use as health resources. State, county, city and municipal health departments also offer useful information. The addresses and phone numbers are in the "Government" section of your phone book.

You can also start a file of stories clipped from local newspapers and magazines. Tape health experts who appear on radio and TV or some of the many excellent full-length shows devoted to health. And if you have access to a computer, you'll find tremendous health resources on the Internet.

You may soon find that the best health expert available is you!

206. Ask Your Doctor about Melatonin

Melatonin may be all you need to fight seasonal affective disorder or "winter blues"; cure insomnia; help you adjust to shift work; or beat jet lag. You can buy it at many health food stores.

A professor of psychiatry, pharmacology and ophthalmology at Oregon Health Sciences University recently reported on his work with melatonin during a meeting of the American Academy of Ophthalmology. The researcher conducted nearly 100 experiments with the substance. The aim of the experiments was to shift the subjects' biological clock backward and forward. As with many things in life, timing was the key to success. To get the desired reaction, melatonin had to be taken at the right time of day. When the timing was right, melatonin was nearly 100 percent effective in resetting a person's biological clock. Travelers and shift workers are among those who may find great benefit in resetting their biological clocks.

The jury is still out on how to take melatonin or how much to take. Ask your doctor what role melatonin may play in keeping you healthy and happy. In the meantime, you can learn more by reading *Melatonin Miracle* by Walter Pierpaoli, M.D.

207. Get an Eye Exam

When was the last time you had your eyes examined?

The American Optometric Association recommends an eye exam every year because your vision can change quickly. You may even be experiencing problems such as recurring headaches that are actually caused by eyestrain. Or you may be developing a problem such as glaucoma—a condition that has no symptoms but results in blindness—without even being aware that something's wrong.

When you schedule your annual physical, make an appointment for an eye exam as well.

208. Cry, Cry, Baby

Research into crying has revealed its many benefits. It helps relieve the physical tension that builds up when you're under stress. And researchers at Cornell University also argue that crying affects the central nervous system, restoring it to a state of balance by easing the stress you feel.

In other words, crying seems to be an emotional safety valve that opens when the inner pressure is too great to handle.

It also seems that all forms of crying are not of equal value in terms of emotional relief. It appears that the chemistry of tears produced when cutting onions is different than that of tears produced by true sorrow.

So next time you feel like crying, yield to nature. Afterward, you'll be glad you did.

209. Groan and Moan

Research shows that groaning is one of the body's natural responses to tension and pain. It relieves physical and emotional stress, sometimes as effectively as medication, meditation or exercise. When you groan, your body vibrates and experiences something like a massage.

Go into a room where you can be comfortable and have privacy. Breathe slowly and deeply. Visualize circumstances that make you feel a strong painful emotion, such as anger, fear or hurt.

As you exhale more deeply, begin to groan. You may feel self-conscious at first, but keep breathing deeply and let the groaning come naturally for ten to fifteen minutes. You'll find that tension gradually fades away.

210. Forgive

Are you harboring a grudge or resentment toward someone? Let it go today and forgive the person. The health benefits of forgiving others—and sometimes of forgiving yourself—are significant. When you forgive a fellow human being, you gain both psychologically and physically.

Research has shown that people become more relaxed when they are forgiving. They also feel physically warmer. Breathing becomes easier, and blood pressure and heart rate lower. In addition, when you forgive another, you connect with the love that is inside you.

Forgiving is simply putting the Golden Rule into practice. Who among us hasn't needed forgiveness? Forgiveness is a way you can let go of anger and pain and increase the love and joy in your life.

211. Take a Calculated Risk

Life is not a dress rehearsal. Playing it safe all the time can reduce the joy of living.

Best-selling author and psychiatrist David Viscott, M.D., believes that if you never reach for the golden ring, you never find out who you really are.

But before making a major life change, ask yourself a few questions: Do you need to make this change? Are you prepared, emotionally and financially? Do you have the support you need from family and friends? Have you made a realistic plan? And a backup plan, in case things don't work out as you intended?

If your answer to these questions is yes, you're probably ready to take a calculated risk. There is the potential for loss when you take a risk—but there's also the potential for gain. Once you've made your decision, go for it and give it your all.

212. Give Yourself Time

In our society, with its instant coffee, instant political polls and instant electronic communication, we are becoming too impatient. Parents, children, spouses, employers and employees all lose patience with each other.

The important things in life—birth, growth, love, friendship, health and healing—all take time and require patience. You can't force a flower to grow, a child to mature, a love to blossom or a wound to heal.

But if you're patient, your life will unfold before you. Maybe not exactly as you had planned or wished it to be, but perhaps even more beautifully than you could have imagined.

When you feel impatient, take a moment to quietly sit and slowly breathe in and out. Let your body relax. The peacefulness that comes with patience will provide a strong foundation for a healthy you.

213. Run for Fun

If you're in good physical shape, running is an excellent activity. You can burn off 600 calories an hour (running at five miles per hour), develop an efficient cardiovascular system, build muscular endurance, enhance muscle strength, and encourage flexibility and coordination.

If running is too difficult for you, brisk walking provides comparable results.

There are other benefits. Local runners' groups provide an opportunity to socialize with men and women who are trying to lead healthy lifestyles. And many races and marathons (and minimarathons) are now dedicated to charitable causes. You can run to keep yourself healthy and, at the same time, help raise funds to fight AIDS, arthritis, cancer or diabetes or to support a local shelter, soup kitchen or nonprofit organization.

But remember: Never start a running or brisk walking program without first checking with your doctor.

214. Instant Calming for Instant Karma

Stress disrupts your normal breathing, reduces the amount of oxygen that reaches your brain and can increase anxiety or panic.

You can combat this response by smiling, maintaining good posture, making a quick mental check for physical tension and keeping your mind clear.

If you smile, even if you feel tense or angry, you will increase the flow of blood and oxygen to your brain. Even just a bit of a smile can effectively begin to reduce your stress level.

Good posture also helps keep your breathing normal and prevents or reduces muscle tension. And by focusing your attention on your body for signs of physical tension, you can take action to release the tense muscle groups. What's more, by letting fearful or angry thoughts go and keeping your mind clear, you will find stress melting away.

215. Open the Door for Stress Relief

Just thirty to sixty seconds in the nearest doorway is all you need to rid yourself of tension.

Whether at home or at work, on an airplane or a train, or in a hotel or a motel on the road, there is a doorway you can use for emergency stress relief.

Stand in the doorway with your forearms against the door frame. Put your right foot out and lean forward. This will stretch the muscles in your shoulders and chest. Next, slide your right foot farther ahead. You will feel a stretch in your calves and hamstrings and around your hips. Finally, while you're leaning forward, use the door frame for support and twist your torso first to one side, then to the other.

Then repeat the exercise with your left foot forward.

This simple stretching routine can relieve muscle tension and stress in less than a minute.

216. Make Friends a Priority

Over the past decade, research studies from around the country, performed by cognitive psychologists such as Martin E. Seligman, Ph.D., have shown that people with close friends become ill less frequently and are better able to fight disease when they do. In addition, they have more *joie de vivre*—the joy of life.

An excellent way to establish friendships is to learn to be a good listener. At some time, everyone needs someone who will listen without judging and without giving unwanted advice.

A second way is to reach out and help someone without waiting to be asked. If a neighbor, a member of your church or synagogue, or a co-worker needs help, make the first move.

A third way is to join a local group that sponsors activities you enjoy such as dancing, bowling or tennis.

217. Write Your Living Will

The first step in creating a living will—a legal document that clearly states your wishes regarding health care treatment—is to empower one person to make your health care decisions for you in case you become incapacitated.

A health care power of attorney can be one of the most important steps you take to safeguard your health. It empowers a specific person (or persons) to make all health decisions for you in case you are unable to do so.

Talk to the person you choose as your health proxy and specifically explain your wishes for the care of your health. If possible, videotape this conversation. It can help avoid conflict later. (If you and your spouse travel together frequently, you may want to consider a third party as an alternate health proxy, in case both of you are injured in an accident.)

A living will with a durable power of attorney and a health care power of attorney can ensure that your health care wishes will be respected. Laws vary from state to state, so check with a lawyer and make sure your doctor has a copy of your health care proxy.

218. Don't Let Downsizing Get You Down

It's only normal to feel anger, loss and even worthlessness when you're downsized out of a job. Work is a central part of most people's lives, emotionally and financially.

Many employment counselors and psychologists have noted that people go through a process of grieving when they lose their jobs. Disbelief is followed by anger, anger by depression and depression, eventually, by acceptance.

Unfortunately, you're more prone to getting sick when under stress—and losing a job is one of the most stressful events in life. So while you go about finding another job, don't forget to eat well and exercise. Many foods contain nutrients that fight depression. And exercise helps your body make endorphins, its own natural antidepressants.

A proper diet and regular exercise will help you stay healthy and active—and ready for that new job when it comes along.

219. Boost Your Brainpower

You probably don't give it much thought, but your brain needs a workout as much as any major muscle group—only giving your brain a regular workout can help boost your creativity and memory.

Mental exercises can be fun, challenging and competitive. Games are a great source of exercise for your mind. Do the crossword puzzle in the paper every day. Or play word games such as Jumble to keep your mind nimble. Checkers, chess and card games such as bridge can add a competitive edge to your mental gymnastics. And these games will also bring you the added benefits of social contact and companionship.

220. Have a Healthy Snack

Some nutritionists counsel against having snacks during the day because most available snack foods are not nutritious and some are even unhealthy for you. But others argue that eating more frequently during the day may actually be better for you.

If you want to snack, keep in mind that all snacks don't have to consist of fattening foods.

You can have an apple or an orange instead of a doughnut. Or you can eat popcorn instead of potato chips. And a slice of vegetarian pizza can be just as tasty as sausage pizza, but it's better for you.

If it helps you feel better during the day, go ahead and snack. But make sure your snacks are nutritious as well as delicious.

221. Grow Healthy with Grains

Grains are perfect as part of a low-fat, high-fiber diet.

Rice, the grain you probably are most familiar with, doesn't come in only two colors—brown and white. There are many delicious kinds of rice available to try, including wild rice and basmati rice. Check a health food store or the ethnic or gourmet foods aisles in the supermarket.

Barley is another choice. Hulled barley is more nutritious than pearled barley and is great as a hot breakfast cereal or side dish or in soups.

The nutty flavor and crunchy texture of buckwheat may also be to your liking. Or you may find that millet—an excellent source of B vitamins and essential minerals—is a welcome addition to your diet. If you're adventurous, look for an ancient Peruvian grain called quinoa (pronounced KEEN-wa) in health food stores.

It's great for a hot breakfast and in puddings, soups and stews.

Creative recipes abound that use these nutritious grains. *Prevention* magazine is an excellent place to find them.

222. Be a Vegetarian—For a Week

Experiment with a vegetarian diet for a week.

True vegetarians (or *vegans*) eat only vegetables. *Lacto-ovo* vegetarians do not eat meat, poultry or fish, but they do eat dairy products and eggs with their veggies. *Semivegetarians* eat little or no red meat, but they do eat some poultry, fish and dairy products.

A strict vegetarian diet reduces your risk of developing some forms of cancer as well as heart disease, adult-onset diabetes, and obesity.

Some strict vegetarians need iron or vitamin B_{12} supplements. If you are seriously considering a long-term switch to one form or another of vegetarianism, talk to your doctor or consult a registered dietitian or nutritionist. You need to make sure your diet includes the protein, carbohydrates, fat, vitamins and minerals that are essential to good health.

223. Be Careful on the Cutting Edge

Use a wooden cutting board. It's healthier.

At first glance, you may think a plastic cutting board would be more sanitary than a wooden one. But researchers at the University of Wisconsin have discovered that wooden cutting boards are better for meats and poultry.

The researchers stored contaminated wooden and plastic cutting boards overnight. Although no one knows why, the wooden boards were completely free of bacteria the next morning, but the plastic ones had higher levels of bacteria.

The researchers also found that the bacteria on some of the wooden boards were dead within three minutes of use. And older wooden cutting boards produced better results than both newer wooden boards and plastic boards.

No matter what kind of cutting board you use, scour it thoroughly with soap and hot water. Avoiding contamination from the microorganisms that live in foods—especially in meats and poultry—can save your life.

224. Be a "Health Food Nut" for a Day

You may laugh when you think of eating what germ, mung beans, alfalfa sprouts and brown rice with seaweed, but you may find them tasty.

Wheat germ can be used to bread fish and meat, or you can sprinkle it on your cereal, mix it in yogurt or add it to your salad. It's rich in vitamin E, several of the B vitamins and zinc—plus it's a great source of protein.

Mung beans and alfalfa sprouts are excellent in salads and stir-fried dishes and on sandwiches. Both foods are rich in many nutrients, especially vitamin C.

Brown rice—which is more nutritious than white rice—is high in fiber and minerals. You can help preserve many of the nutrients that are lost in cooking by soaking the rice for forty-five minutes and then cooking it in that water.

Give this "health food" a try. You may be surprised at how good it tastes.

225. Aim for Your Target Heart Rate

Learn how to determine what your heart rate should be during aerobic exercise. Exercise physiologists have determined how long your heart has to beat at a certain rate for you to benefit from your exercise.

To get the most benefit from aerobic exercise, for example, your heart should stay within what is called your training zone. The

American College of Sports Medicine and other fitness groups use a standard formula to determine what a person's training zone is: Simply subtract your age from 220. Multiply that number by 0.6 to find the low end of your training zone. Multiply it by 0.85 to find the high end of your training zone.

During exercise, take a moment to find your pulse. Using the second hand on your watch, count the number of pulses in one minute (or count your pulse in ten seconds and multiply by six). This is your heart rate. Compare your heart rate with your training zone. If you're at the beginning or end of your workout, your heart rate should be at the low end of your training zone. If you're at the height of your workout, it should be at the high end. If your heart rate is higher than your training zone, you're exercising too hard. If it's lower, you're not working hard enough to really benefit from the exercise.

226. Warm Up, Cool Down

Warm up with a few careful stretches before you begin to perform any exercise.

Stretching is vital because it helps prevent injuries. When you start stretching your muscles, you will feel some strain, but you shouldn't feel any pain. Slow and steady stretching for five to ten minutes is best for your body.

After you complete your exercise, you need a period in which to cool down while your heart rate returns to normal. Stretching again after a workout can provide a good cooldown and reduce the intensity of any muscle aches you may feel the next day. And a massage after your workout can stimulate your circulation and help rid your muscles of the waste products that build up while you exercise.

227. Give Yourself a Helping Hand

If you work with your hands all day—especially at a keyboard—they may get stiff and tense after hours of work. But you can easily relax them in only a few minutes.

Try massaging the front and back of your right hand with the thumb and fingers of your left hand. Gently massage the palm of your hand with your thumb and the back of your hand with your fingers. Now use your right hand to massage your left.

Another stress buster involves grasping the four fingers of one hand with the other and gently bending your hand back at the wrist, holding them in that position for about five seconds.

Making a tight fist and then opening and closing your hand a number of times also relieves hand tension.

228. Create Your Own Dance Studio at Home

You don't need to go to a dance class or dance studio to get the aerobic benefits of dancing. You can create a dance studio in the comfort of your own home.

Dancing burns up a lot of calories and is a great way to lose weight and keep it off. Dancing also pumps oxygen throughout your body, leaving you energized long after your dancing is done.

Start with nonimpact or low-impact aerobic dancing at home. These activities don't require any jumping, and your feet are kept close to the floor. You can get a brisk workout with minimal risk of injury.

Roll up the carpet, put on your favorite beat and dance your way to health and renewed energy.

229. Jump for Joy

You probably haven't jumped rope since you were a child. But jumping is a rigorous activity, which is why boxers use it in training.

The first thing you need, of course, is a rope. You can buy a jump rope, but a piece of old clothesline is really all you need. If you're standing with it under both feet, the ends of the rope should reach to your armpits on both sides.

Jump slowly until you find your rhythm. Pace yourself so that you jump smoothly. You may find jumping tiring, so jump for a minute or two and then rest. Fifteen minutes of jumping rope will give you a good workout.

As you progress, you can jump longer and faster and even throw in some fancy footwork. And you may soon find that jumping is no chore—and that you're jumping just for the joy of it, just as you did in childhood.

230. Walk in Water

A walk in water can do wonders for your health!

Water walking was first developed to help people with injuries exercise. But it wasn't long before experts in rehabilitative therapy saw that this exercise could be of benefit to everyone.

You can get your exercise by walking in water in a pool, a lake or the ocean. The water can be only up to your ankles or as high as your calves.

If you water walk at a steady pace, you can burn off 300–500 calories an hour. And because you have to overcome the water's resistance, water walking at two miles an hour gives you the same benefit as walking on land at three miles an hour. Of course, if you walk in shallow water, which has less resistance, you'll need to walk faster than in deeper water.

During the warmer months, or any time in an indoor pool, water walking can be an enjoyable variation in your regular exercise schedule.

231. Try an Anti-aging "Pill"

Exercise is probably the world's greatest medicine. It reduces stress, anxiety and depression and can help prevent heart disease and other illnesses. A recent report from the National Institute on Aging notes that "if exercise could be packed in a pill, it would be the single most widely prescribed and beneficial medicine in the nation." In fact, regular exercise may prevent most age-related physical deterioration. (Look at Jack LaLanne—he's in his eighties, yet he's as fit as a much younger man.)

Researchers at the University of Florida Center for Exercise Sciences have studied the anti-aging effects of exercise. And they have found that seniors benefit from regular exercise more than any other age group. In fact, even men and women in their nineties achieve great benefits from beginning regular exercise.

No matter how old or young you are, it's never too late or too soon to begin exercising.

232. Relax Body and Mind with a Winter Workout

Get the physical exercise you need and the mental relaxation you crave by taking up cross-country skiing.

Cross-country skiing—also called Nordic skiing—exercises all the major muscle groups in your body. It's one of the best aerobic exercises there is.

If you think you'd enjoy this activity, consider taking lessons to start. You'll need to learn how to use your poles and how to maneuver across the terrain on your skis. You don't need to purchase expensive equipment to get started. Everything you need can be rented at a reasonable cost from your local sporting goods store.

Dress warmly, using layering to keep out the cold and wick away sweat. Wear waterproof clothing as an outer layer, always wear a hat and don't forget sunglasses to protect your eyes from the sun glaring off the snow, and sunscreen for exposed skin.

Once you try cross-country skiing, you may never want to come in from the cold again!

233. Soothe Sore Feet

Tired, sore feet will respond to a soothing bath with warm water and footbath salts. The salts contain alkali, which will also soften your skin as well as provide cleansing action.

You can also put a little lemon juice in lukewarm water to soak away aches. Lavender oil, Burow's solution (which comes as a powder to mix with water) and cider vinegar can also help relieve the pain of sore feet.

You may also want to soak your feet in cold water for fifteen minutes twice a day if they are irritated by the materials in your socks or shoes.

234. Take a Child's-Eye View of the World

Get down on your hands and knees to see what a child sees and get a realistic view of how to make your home safe for children.

For starters, install safety plugs in all electrical outlets that a child can reach. Put covers over all radiators and other sources of home heating and make sure you have window guards. Keep beds, desks, tables and chairs away from windows, so children can't climb up and out.

Go through your home from room to room and look at it from a child's viewpoint. You'll be amazed at what potential hazards you find—from the ant trap behind the stove to the sweet and deadly antifreeze in the garage.

235. Install a Carbon Monoxide Detector

Sometimes it may seem as if the whole family has come down with the flu and just can't shake it. Or perhaps one of the children seems to be listless and fatigued for no obvious reason. It may even appear that a parent or child is suffering from depression.

Yet the real cause of these "illnesses" may be carbon monoxide poisoning, and the solution to your problem could be a carbon monoxide detector.

These devices are inexpensive and as easy to install as a smoke detector. Some are battery-operated, some are hardwired into your home's circuitry, and some offer a combination of power sources. (Researchers at *Consumer Reports* prefer the hardwired models.)

First Alert and other well-known companies now make carbon monoxide detectors. If you buy one, make sure it is marked as meeting the new UL safety standard: UL#2034. For more information, contact the Consumer Product Safety Commission in Washington, D.C., at 1-800-638-2772.

236. Clean Air Naturally

Indoor air pollution can be reduced by common houseplants.

A good rule of thumb is to have a least one plant for every 100 square feet in the room. To be effective, the plants themselves must be healthy, so give them enough light and water. Avoid over-watering, which can cause mold or mildew to grow.

The pollution-fighting power of plants may lie in their root systems and the microorganisms in the soil. By cutting back lower branches, you expose the soil to air and increase your plant's effectiveness at cleaning it.

Ask your local nursery about which plants are best. Corn and spider plants, philodendrons, ferns and dracaena are among those frequently suggested.

237. Reduce Your Exposure to Electromagnetic Radiation

Although the final answers are not yet in regarding the health effects of exposure to electromagnetic radiation, it is better to err on the side of safety. Many population studies link exposure to electromagnetic fields given off by electrical power lines and electrical appliances to brain tumors, leukemia and other cancers.

You can take a few simple steps to reduce unnecessary exposure until we know more about this controversial subject.

When you are not using electrical appliances, keep them unplugged. Some appliances give off low-frequency electromagnetic radiation when plugged in even though they are turned off. And use regular tungsten lightbulbs. They cost more to run than fluorescent lights, but they give off less electromagnetic radiation.

And if you have a microwave, have it checked by a repairperson each year to make sure the seals are still tight.

238. Get the Lead Out

Lead in your drinking water usually comes from an aging municipal water system or from the plumbing in your own home.

If you suspect there's a problem, call your local office of the Environmental Protection Agency for information about testing your water. Due to the growing awareness of lead in drinking water, many municipalities are now offering free or low-cost lead testing. Usually, they'll ask you to submit two water samples: one taken when you haven't run the tap for a few hours, and the other after you've let the water run for several minutes.

Until the results of these tests are known, use bottled water.

239. Make a Fire Plan

Plan what you'll do in case of a fire—and make sure everyone in your family also knows what they're supposed to do.

Then walk through the planned escape route from each room in your house. Make sure that doors are not blocked by any obstacles and that windows are not permanently locked for "safety."

As part of your fire safety plan, pick a spot outside your home where everyone will meet immediately after escaping the fire. This will allow you to make sure that everyone has made it out safely.

If your home has a second or third floor, think about buying portable escape ladders and practice using them.

You may want to have a surprise fire drill at night, because that's when most fires occur. Many people die unnecessarily in fires because they didn't plan ahead. Take steps now to make sure that doesn't happen to your family.

240. Check Your Smoke Detector

Don't think your job is done just because you've installed smoke detectors around your home. You need to check them every few weeks to make sure that they'll work when you need them.

You also need to keep your smoke detectors clean. Dust and spiderwebs can interfere with their sensors. So can paint, so don't paint a smoke detector to make it more aesthetically pleasing. And don't forget to change batteries according to the manufacturer's instructions. Some people change the batteries once a year when they change their clocks from standard to daylight saving time. Whatever your method, make a plan and stick to it. Smoke detectors save lives, but only if you give them the power to.

241. Be a Survivor

Many parts of the country can be hit by earthquakes, floods, wildfires, tornadoes, hurricanes, blizzards and other natural disasters.

If you live in an area where one of these things can happen to you, stock your home with enough supplies so that you can survive for at least four days.

Water should be at the top of your supply list. Keep at least three gallons of water per person, stored in clean, durable plastic containers. You should also stock a battery-operated radio (with extra batteries), battery-operated flashlights, candles, canned or dried foods, juices and a can opener. You will also need a well-stocked first aid kit and any medications that you or a family member might need.

Every month, replace the water and check on any other items that can become outdated.

It may seem like a lot of work—but if disaster strikes, you'll be a survivor.

242. Exercise without Getting Out of Your Seat

You can fight stiffness and fatigue with a few simple exercises no matter where you are.

For example, sit up straight with your feet flat on the floor. Tense your neck and shoulder muscles for five seconds, then relax. Make fists and tense the muscles in your arms, then relax. You can do this with all the major muscle groups in your body and get rid of any tension—while you remain seated!

You can also perform flexibility exercises in a chair, such as wiggling your toes, bending and straightening your knees, reaching upward with your arms and simply shrugging your shoulders.

These simple exercises can keep you from getting tired and listless. They may even make you feel refreshed and reinvigorated.

243. Travel with a Medicine Kit

Take a well-stocked medicine kit with you when you travel.
A medicine kit can not only help keep you comfortable should

you come down with a minor illness on your trip. It may even save your life.

You should use a waterproof container, preferably made of clear plastic (to help you find things more easily). If you take medication regularly, keep the amount you expect to use in the medicine kit and at least an equal amount in another bag—just in case you lose the kit. Also, ask your doctor for extra prescriptions.

Your medicine travel kit should include over-the-counter painkillers (such as aspirin, ibuprofen and acetaminophen), antacids, antibiotics, antihistamines, antiseptics, bandages, adhesive tape, gauze, decongestants, antidiarrheal medicines, feminine hygiene products, motion sickness pills, tweezers, a pocket knife and a thermometer.

244. Choose Your Pharmacist Wisely

One of the most important services that a pharmacist can provide is to maintain a profile of the drugs you're taking. If you're taking a number of different medicines, this record can literally save your life. Because although some medications may be perfectly safe when taken individually, they are lethal in combination. With all the specialists we all see, one doctor may not realize how many drugs you're taking. But your pharmacist—if he keeps a profile—would see any dangerous mix and warn you.

A good pharmacist will also take the time to answer your questions about medications you're taking. And he or she can sometimes suggest generic or even over-the-counter alternatives to expensive brand-name prescription drugs.

At a time when fewer people have personal physicians, a pharmacist who knows you can be a godsend.

245. Have a Cranberry on the Rocks

Each year, about 20 percent of American women and 5 percent of American men get urinary tract infections. Over the years, doctors have debated whether or not cranberry juice helps to fight these infections.

No one knows for sure whether or not it does, but if you'd like to see for yourself, drink at least ten glasses of water and one glass of cranberry juice each day. The theory is that the fluid will wash the bacteria out of your bladder. And it may. A recent study found that four to six ounces of cranberry juice every day prevented recurring infections in high-risk patients.

246. Try the Newest Aphrodisiac

If you're no longer interested in sex, the antidepressant Wellbutrin may help you more than ginseng, oysters or any of the other well-known substances touted as aphrodisiacs.

Researchers at a sex therapy center found that Wellbutrin had a positive effect on the sex drives of both men and women. This came as quite a surprise because most antidepressant drugs have adverse effects on the libido.

Scientists are not sure exactly why the drug has this effect and whether it is acting physiologically or psychologically on the individuals who take it. Wellbutrin stimulates the production of dopamine, which affects many aspects of body functioning, including sexuality.

Talk to your doctor about Wellbutrin if you think it may be of help to you.

247. Stay Sober for Sailing

According to a report in the *Journal of the American Medical Association*, mixing alcohol with water activities can be lethal.

More than 50 percent of the people who die in boating accidents on weekends are legally drunk. And about half of the time, deaths occur in boats that are anchored or drifting.

If you go out boating, you can't assume it's safe to drink even if you're just along for the ride. There is no "designated captain" who can stay sober so that you can drink.

Most of the time, the captain or the operator of the boat plays no role at all in the fatalities that occur.

Enjoy sailing on the ocean or a lake—but be sure to leave the booze behind.

248. Watch *When* You Eat

In terms of diet and heart disease, when you eat may be as important as what you eat.

A researcher at Boston University School of Medicine discovered that the French have half the death rate from heart disease of Americans. And when the researcher looked at the eating habits of a group of working-class Parisians, he found that they consumed 57 percent of their calories before 2 P.M.

In contrast, Americans consumed only 38 percent of their calories by midafternoon.

The report to the American Heart Association suggested that because the French were active for a longer period of time after their biggest meal, fewer calories were stored as fat. But because Americans were more sedentary after their biggest meal, the extra calories became stored as fat, putting Americans at higher risk for heart disease.

249. Eat a Healthy Breakfast

All the research to date suggests that your mood, your ability to think clearly and your energy level are all positively affected by eating a good breakfast, according to the American Dietetic

Association and other nutritional groups. A healthy meal in the morning also makes your body better able to withstand the stresses that come your way each day.

If mornings are hard for you, try planning your breakfast the night before. There is no special "breakfast food" that you need to eat. Fruit, low-fat cheese, yogurt, cereal and wheat germ are all good choices.

The traditional high-fat, high-cholesterol American breakfast (such as eggs, bacon, and fatty buttered muffins) is best avoided.

Get up, get a good breakfast, and get going!

250. Get Out of Your Rut

You don't need to make big changes to get out of a rut or to put some pizzazz back into your daily life. Sometimes you just need to fine-tune the little things.

Be spontaneous. One night, surprise your spouse by taking him or her out to a special dinner at the best restaurant in town. (You may have to save up to do this, but that can be part of the fun.)

Or vary the way that you go to work. If you drive every day but can take mass transit, use it one day and let someone else fight rush-hour traffic while you read a good book or sit back and enjoy the scenery.

Analyze your daily behavior to see what repetitive patterns you've fallen into. Then make a few easy changes. You may find your life to be more invigorating as a result.

251. Iron Things Out

If you are listless and pale, you may be suffering from iron-deficiency anemia. While only 2 percent of American men are affected, according to the United States government, most premenopausal women in America do not take in as much iron as they need. Menstruation, pregnancy and breast-feeding make the problem worse.

If you are suffering because of an inadequate supply of iron, don't worry. It's easy to correct. The Daily Value for iron is only eighteen milligrams. Lean red meats, green leafy vegetables, wheat germ and foods fortified with iron can all help restore your health.

Or talk to your doctor about using iron supplements. If you decide to take them, keep in mind that you will absorb more iron if you take the supplement on an empty stomach. Since this can cause upset stomach in some people, however, you may prefer to take iron supplements with meals.

252. Explain Your Pain

Pain is a sign that something is wrong. But for your doctor to help you, he or she has to find out what kind of pain you are experiencing.

Tell your doctor whether your pain is throbbing, burning, sharp, dull, shooting or pulsing. And let your doctor know when the pain began. Was it after exercising? After climbing two flights of stairs? After eating?

If you've taken anything for your pain, let your doctor know whether it gave you relief. It is also important to tell the doctor if your pain seems to move from one area of your body to another or if it comes and goes.

The more you can tell your physician, the easier it will be to diagnose your problem. Before you see your doctor, write down as much information as you can. We all forget things because of the stress we feel in a doctor's office.

253. Learn Cancer's Warning Signs

Cancer may be 100 different diseases with a wide variety of causes, but you need to learn what the major warning symptoms are. Early detection is the key to successful treatment and survival.

It is currently estimated that three of ten Americans alive today will get cancer. The most common forms of the disease are lung cancer, colon and rectal cancer, breast cancer, prostate cancer, cancer of the urinary tract and uterine cancer.

According to the American Cancer Society, the major warning signs are:

- A change in bowel or bladder habits
- A lump or thickening in the breast or another body part
- A noticeable change in a wart or mole
- A sore throat that lingers
- Difficulty swallowing
- Unusual vaginal or rectal bleeding

If you have any of these symptoms, see your physician as soon as possible.

254. Learn the Warning Signs of Diabetes

There are two kinds of diabetes. The more severe form is known as Type I, which usually occurs before age forty and is treated with insulin injections. Type II diabetes usually begins after age forty. People who are overweight are at risk. Frequently, diet and exercise alone can control this form of the disease.

Early diagnosis of diabetes is critical. It's easy to learn the warning signs of diabetes if you remember the acronyms CAUTION and DIABETES.

Constant urination	Drowsiness
Abnormal thirst	Itching
Unusual hunger	A family history of diabetes
The rapid loss of weight	Blurred vision
Irritability	Excessive weight
Obvious weakness and fatigue	Tingling, numbness or pain
Nausea and vomiting	in the extremities
	Easy fatigue
	Skin infection or slow healing
	cuts, especially on the feet

If you have some of these symptoms, make an appointment

with your doctor. A simple blood test will reveal whether or not you have diabetes.

255. Discourage Gallstones

More than sixteen million Americans, mostly women, get gallstones, and many experience severe pain. Sometimes surgery is even required.

The most common kind of gallstone is made of cholesterol—the same fat that can clog your arteries and cause heart disease. A genetic error in cholesterol metabolism may make certain people more susceptible to gallstone formation. Being female, obese, diabetic or having a family history of gallstones are all major risk factors that increase your chances of getting them.

You can't do much about your family or your gender, but you can reduce your risk of developing this potentially serious problem by eating a diet that is rich in fiber (foods such as fresh vegetables and fruits and whole grains), consuming less dietary fat and avoiding foods that are high in sugar or refined carbohydrates.

256. Fight Gout

A gout attack—with pain in your big toe, heel, ankle, wrist or elbow—can last for hours or for a few excruciating days. The attack can be set off by drinking beer or wine, eating a diet rich in red meats or organ meats, eating sardines or anchovies or taking certain medicines (such as diuretics).

Gout is actually a form of arthritis and is caused by high levels of uric acid in the blood. The acid can form into sharp crystals that collect in the joints, causing inflammation and pain.

Prescription drugs such as colchicine—and even some over-the-counter drugs such as ibuprofen—can bring immediate relief.

Prevent gout by cutting back on red meats and alcohol, losing excess weight and taking any medication your doctor prescribes.

257. Take Your Blood Pressure Twice

Your blood pressure is measured using two numbers. The first measures what is called systolic pressure, meaning the pressure exerted against the walls of your arteries while your heart is beating. The second measures what is called diastolic pressure, or the pressure between heartbeats when your heart is at rest.

The two numbers are recorded one over the other, as in 120/80. Normal blood pressure is around 139/84. Mild high blood pressure runs from 140/90.

You need two or more readings, taken on separate occasions, to get an accurate blood pressure measurement.

You should also have your blood pressure taken when standing, seated and lying down, since this will give your doctor a better idea of what's normal for you. Have your blood pressure checked annually. Keeping your blood pressure normal will reduce your risk of heart attack, stroke and kidney disease.

258. Know the Risks of Getting Pneumonia

Once called the old person's friend, pneumonia is the sixth leading cause of death in the United States. Although the disease is caused by various bacteria, viruses, toxins and fungi, its risk factors include advanced age, smoking, alcoholism, recent hospitalization, poor nutrition, a cold, emphysema, chronic bronchitis, sickle-cell anemia and taking immune-suppressing drugs.

If you have a chest cold that worsens, see your doctor and take the medication he prescribes. Get plenty of rest, use a cool-mist humidifier in your room and do not use any cough suppressants.

259. Don't Give Aspirin to a Child with a Fever

Never give aspirin to a child under the age of nineteen who appears to have symptoms of a cold, the flu or chicken pox. Use acetaminophen or nothing at all.

A deadly health problem, Reye's syndrome, is associated with aspirin use in children with the flu or chicken pox. Because it is difficult for a parent or adult caregiver to know the cause of a child's aches, pains and fever, it is important not to take any risks.

Reye's syndrome can produce serious damage to the brain and liver. At first, the flu or chicken pox may seem to be going away. But then persistent vomiting, confusion, extreme fatigue, seizures and personality changes set in. If the condition goes untreated, coma and even death can occur.

The safest course of action is to not give children aspirin if they have a fever. This will prevent Reye's syndrome from occurring.

260. Stay Out of D-A-N-G-E-R

Learn the meaning of DANGER, an acronym devised to help you remember the warning signals of stroke. The signs are:

Dizziness

Absentmindedness or temporary memory loss

Numbness or weakness in the arm, leg or face

Garbled speech

Eye problems (such as double vision or temporary loss of sight)

Recent onset of severe headaches

Learning these warning signs will tell you when to get immediate medical attention. Stroke is the third leading cause of death in the United States, and by recognizing an important warning signal, you can reduce your risk of serious brain damage, crippling and even premature death.

261. Test Your Heart

If you're at risk for heart disease, think about getting an exercise stress test. This test measures how well your heart holds up under physical exertion. The results will let you and your doctor know what exercises you can do safely and how intensely you can plan to exercise.

Should you have this test? Only your doctor can say. But the answer may be yes if you smoke, are over age forty-five, don't exercise or have diabetes, a family history of heart disease or chest pains when you do exercise.

Talk to your doctor about the benefits of having this test. It may be the first step you need toward a healthier lifestyle.

262. Get Up and Get Going

Exercise is a great way to start your day. It helps get the juices flowing and stimulates the production of endorphins, your body's natural opiates.

But early-morning exercise may confer other benefits as well. Researchers at an Arizona health institute conducted a study that revealed that people who exercised in the morning were more likely to stick with their daily workouts than people who worked out later.

The scientists reported that 75 percent of those who exercised in the morning were still doing so one year later. In contrast, only 50 percent of those who exercised in the middle of the day were still active. And only 25 percent of those who exercised in the evening were still working out.

If you have a hard time getting motivated in the morning, lay out your workout clothes next to your bed the night before, so they are the first things you see when you wake up in the morning. Once you discover the benefits of exercising in the morning, you'll look forward to your A.M. workout.

263. Snuff Out Smokeless Tobacco

Cigarette smoking has declined dramatically in the past twenty years, but the use of smokeless tobacco is up significantly. Dipping snuff has increased the most sharply.

Many people erroneously believe that smokeless tobacco is safe. In reality, it increases the risk of developing oral cancer and other health problems.

Men who use smokeless tobacco have nearly four times the risk of developing oral cancer of those who don't use it, according to the American Cancer Society. The results of a study of women showed similar results. Smokeless tobacco can also cause gum and periodontal disease, contribute to heart disease and high blood pressure, stimulate the development of benign but painful oral lesions and harm the fetus in a pregnant woman. And the nicotine in snuff is just as addictive as the nicotine in cigarettes.

Call your local chapter of the American Cancer Society for information on how to kick the habit.

264. Base Your Exercise on Body Type

Exercise can do wonders for your health and energy level but it can't change your body type. And your body type may make some activities easier and more effective for you. Are you an endomorph, a mesomorph or an ectomorph? Most people fall into one of these body-type categories, based on height, build, muscle tone and distribution of body fat.

In general, endomorphs are small-boned, chubby, not muscular, and broader at the hips than shoulders. Mesomorphs are usually rugged, big-boned, muscular and broad-shouldered. And ectomorphs have narrow shoulders, chests and hips, long arms and legs, and little body fat.

If you are an endomorph, you may benefit most from nonimpact or low-impact aerobic activities such as bike riding, swimming and brisk walking. Walking, running, martial arts and sports such as tennis may benefit mesomorphs the most. And for ectomorphs, tennis, basketball, racquet sports, jogging and other similar exercises may bring the biggest aerobic benefits.

Consider using your body type as a guide when choosing how to exercise.

265. Keep Cool When It's Hot

If you choose to exercise outside when it's hot, use common sense. Wear loose, lightweight clothing that allows you to perspire freely. Exercise more moderately—and don't push for a personal best. Work out in the early morning or near sunset, when it is cooler. And drink water even if you don't feel thirsty. Some exercise experts suggest that you drink about ten ounces of water fifteen minutes or so before you begin exercising. And drink water during your workout to replenish the fluids you lose.

A little forethought and common sense will save you unnecessary problems.

266. Calm Colic

Researchers in Israel were able to reduce colic in half of the infants who were given an herbal tea as part of their study. The tea contained chamomile, licorice, fennel and balm-mint. The babies were given this mixture after every attack of colic for a week. Another group of babies—the control group—was given a drink that smelled and looked like the herbal tea but did not contain any of the healing herbs. There was no reduction in colic in this group.

These herbs have been known to prevent spasms in adults. The herb mixture that the researchers used is available commercially in Italy. The researchers believe that the mixture relaxes the stomach and relieves intestinal cramps.

If your baby suffers from colic and nothing seems to be working, both you and your baby may find relief from a calming herbal tea. Talk to your pediatrician and remember to cool the tea before giving it to your baby.

267. Don't Apologize for Eating Beans

Soaking beans and other legumes in water for twelve hours before cooking them can limit their gaseous side effects, according to researchers in Spain.

Soaking the beans before cooking reduced the sugar content of the beans by up to 30 percent—it's the sugar that causes flatulence. Boiling was more effective than using a pressure cooker in reducing gas from kidney beans, while lentils did better in a pressure cooker. Chickpeas and kidney beans that were kept in their cooking water for five hours at a temperature of ninety-five degrees Fahrenheit had even less sugar.

Beans play an important role in reducing your risk of colon cancer and heart disease, but not everyone needs to know when you've eaten them!

268. Do Some Heavy-Lifting Housework

Researchers at the Mayo Clinic in Rochester, Minnesota, have released the results of a recent study that shows that women who run, swim and perform aerobic exercises such as dancing have less back strength than homemakers. Homemakers who carry their babies and lift heavy loads of wet laundry day after day appear to be more fit then their aerobicizing sisters.

The researchers' results show that the homemakers had more upper-body and arm strength. This is usually associated with back strength from weight-bearing exercises. (You can be aerobically fit and yet not be strong.) The homemakers' heavy-lifting housework decreases their risk of developing osteoporosis.

So in addition to going to the gym or exercising at home in

front of an exercise video, lift that laundry and tote those groceries with gusto!

269. Limit TV Time

Watching too much television keeps kids from being active and increases the chances that they'll become overweight. According to a study conducted at Boston University School of Medicine, less active children were three times more likely than more physically active children to be overweight. In fact, by age seven those children who watched more TV had a measurable increase in fat for every *hour* of TV they watched each day. Sadly, many of these youngsters seemed to already be full-grown couch potatoes at the tender age of seven or eight.

Be a good role model for your kids by exercising with them. And encourage them to participate in physical activities at school and in local neighborhood groups. TV alone doesn't make kids fat, but a less active lifestyle sure does.

270. Set Up a Twenty-Four-Hour Health Club at Home

The Cable Health Club provides twenty-four-hour programming on health topics such as aerobics, equipment training, recreational sports techniques, personal grooming, and product news. The cable channel also offers news updates on hot topics in health and nutrition, has a home-shopping segment and offers valuable tips on ordering healthy foods when eating out and on making delicious low-calorie recipes at home.

About 2.5 million Americans can get Cable Health Club via cable TV; another 3.5 million can get the show via satellite. If this show is not available in your area, call your local cable company. You may be able to receive the channel on request—and at no extra charge.

271. Get Down on Your Knees

Psychologists at Rutgers University studied almost 3,000 people who regularly attended church or synagogue. The scientists found that religious faith and involvement in a church enhanced these people's lives. The participants in the study seemed to be more emotionally and physically fit and better able to live on their own than people for whom religion was not important. In addition, the researchers found that even men who were housebound suffered significantly less depression if they had strong religious beliefs.

The social support these individuals received from members of their congregations played an important role in enhancing their lives. But that is not the whole story. It seems that deep inner spirituality plays an important role in promoting and sustaining life.

272. Be Flexible and Live to Be 100

Researchers have found that people who live to be 100 seem to have a number of personality traits in common. And all of these traits can be described by one word: flexibility.

Individuals who reach the century mark respond creatively to change, control their anxiety, integrate new ideas into their lives, and remain flexible and adaptable. And maybe most importantly, people who make it to 100 years of age really want to get there.

273. Eat Cheaply and Eat Well

A healthy diet can be as good for your budget as it is for your body. Researchers at Pennsylvania State University and at the Bassett Hospital Research Institute in Cooperstown, New York, studied the eating habits of about 300 people. All the participants in the study lived in rural areas and had high cholesterol levels. The researchers devised healthy eating plans for the participants.

When they later reviewed the participants' eating habits, the scientists found that the people who were most successful in lowering their blood cholesterol levels also spent less money on food than they had previously.

Many people mistakenly believe that in order to eat healthy and nutritious foods, they have to pay through the nose. Actually, most of the foods that are good for you—fresh vegetables and fruits, whole grains and beans—are quite inexpensive. In fact, they cost a lot less than meats, cheeses and processed foods.

274. Make Sure Your Medicine Is Gender-Specific

Many women may need to take one-third less of certain drugs than their doctors prescribe for them, according to a report delivered at a meeting of the American Women's Medical Association. Why?

Recent research indicates that women have higher brain blood flow and slower gastric processes than men, which necessitate different drug doses.

Gender differences are extremely significant in terms of drug use. Women of reproductive age have a higher incidence of adverse drug reactions than men of the same age. And women experience twice as many deaths from adverse drug reactions as do men.

If you are taking medication and it doesn't seem to be working as intended, talk to your doctor. You may need to have the dosage adjusted or switch to a different drug.

275. Watch Out for "Switched" Drugs

Aleve, Pepcid AC and Tagamet HB are just three of the scores of powerful prescription drugs that you can now buy right off the shelf at the pharmacy. But these new "switched" products are being recommended for the treatment of different health problems than their prescription versions.

Aleve is recommended for the treatment of muscle aches and pains, for example. But as a prescription drug, it is known as Naprosyn or Anaprox and is used to treat arthritis. Tagamet HB and Pepcid AC are recommended for heartburn, but as prescription drugs they are used to treat ulcers.

The FDA is considering approving drug switching for about seventy prescription products. Many health experts are concerned that this could result in a dramatic increase in drug accidents. Switched drugs can interact with one another, and with prescription drugs, in ways that may be detrimental to your health.

Make sure your doctor knows what drugs you're taking—and make sure your pharmacist notes all the medications you use in his or her records.

276. Choose the Cheapest Painkiller

Nonsteroidal anti-inflammatory drugs (NSAIDs) such as aspirin and ibuprofen are all pretty similar in terms of safety and effectiveness, according to a recent report in the *Archives of Internal Medicine*. Yet each advertiser claims that his product is less toxic and has fewer side effects than the other guy's.

Researchers have found that tests of these painkillers, which were paid for by the drug manufacturers, always supported the claims of whoever paid for the studies. Of sixty-one studies that the researchers looked at, fifty-six found that the drug made by the company that paid for the study was the superior drug.

Be a smart consumer. When you're in a drugstore or pharmacy, check the prices on the bottles of aspirin, acetaminophen, ibuprofen and naproxen sodium before you buy. And make your choice based on the price, not the hype.

277. Hold the Whole Milk

Young children get more fat and saturated fat than they should, according to the U.S. Department of Agriculture, and 75 percent get more cholesterol than they need.

A recent study published in the *American Journal of Public Health* advocated low-fat dairy products for even young children. According to this report, kids get 11 percent of their total fat and 18 percent of their saturated fat each day from whole milk. About 40 percent of children's daily dietary cholesterol comes from a combination of whole milk and eggs.

You can help keep your children healthy by serving them low-fat or skim milk at home. Then talk to the people responsible for lunches at your child's school. Many school lunch programs provide whole milk to children, instead of the healthier low-fat or skim milk. See if you can get them to make a healthier choice.

278. Check with Your Doctor about Cholesterol

The National Cholesterol Education Program recommends cholesterol tests for all adults over age twenty. But a recent report published in the *Journal of the American Medical Association* suggests that routine cholesterol testing may not be necessary until after age thirty-five.

In the report, researchers from the University of California, San Francisco, argue that cholesterol intervention in low-risk adults and in people with high cholesterol levels but no other heart disease risk factors has little benefit.

In fact, the researchers claim that cholesterol intervention in low-risk adults may do more harm than good—and that cholesterol intervention to prevent heart disease appears to be effective even if it isn't begun until middle age.

Talk to your doctor about when to get a cholesterol test.

279. Monitor Cholesterol Drugs

Make sure you know the latest information on any medication you're taking to lower cholesterol levels. Recently, serious questions have been raised about the safety of two classes of cholesterol-lowering drugs: the fibrates and the statins.

Lopid (or gemfibrozil) and Atromid-S (or clofibrate) are two fibrates involved. And Mevacor (lovastatin), Pravachol (pravastatin), Zocor (simvastatin) and Lescol (fluvastatin) are four of the statins in question.

In a report in the *Journal of the American Medical Association*, two researchers from the University of California, San Francisco, claim that these two classes of drugs, used by tens of millions of Americans, may cause cancer in some people.

The researchers are not concerned about the effects of these drugs on people with heart disease or at high risk for heart disease, but they are concerned about people who start the drugs in their twenties, then stay on them for life. For people who need long-term drug therapy, the researchers feel that two other kinds of drugs are better: cholestyramine (Cholybar, Questran, Questran Light) and the vitamin niacin (Nicobid).

If you're taking cholesterol-lowering drugs, discuss them with your doctor from time to time to keep abreast of new information about these potent chemicals.

280. Beware of "Beauty Parlor Stroke"

The design of shampoo sinks in beauty parlors may cause strokes in older women, according to a neurologist at New York Medical College, who first reported this phenomenon in 1992. Women in beauty parlors are forced to hyperextend their necks while having their hair washed in the sink. This causes a partial shutdown of blood flow to the brain. In four of the five cases studied by the neurologist, the women suffered actual brain damage and stroke symptoms that did not go away.

His conclusions?

In a letter published in the *Journal of the American Medical Association*, the doctor recommends that beauty parlors modify their sinks for older folks. In addition, he advises any elderly person to think twice about daily activities that require stretching the neck and/or hanging the head for any length of time.

281. Air-Bag It

Make sure that the next car you buy comes with air bags.

Researchers analyzed information from all over the country about automobile accidents in the years 1985–91 to determine what effect air bags had on automobile fatalities. The researchers published their results in the *American Journal of Public Health*. The results showed a 28 percent reduction in driver deaths from frontal crashes in cars with air bags. There was even a 31 percent reduction in mortality among drivers of cars with air bags who did not use their seat belts.

The benefits gained by having an air bag were even higher in large cars. Fatalities in bigger vehicles were reduced by as much as 49 percent. They came to the conclusion that if all passenger vehicles were equipped with air bags, at least on the driver's side, about 4,000 lives could be saved in just one year.

282. Get the Most from Your Produce

To keep valuable nutrients at peak levels in produce, pick vegetables that are crisp and firm and avoid soft, bruised produce. And since fruits and vegetables will spoil quickly if left at room temperature, keep them refrigerated. If you have limited storage room in your refrigerator, make it a habit to stop by the produce market every day or two. Your increased health and vitality will make it worth the effort.

283. Adopt an Eskimo Diet

A study looking for a link between Eskimos and their low incidence of heart disease focused attention on the Eskimo diet, which is rich in fish.

The study indicated that the cold-water fish Eskimos eat protects them against cardiovascular disease. Cold-water fish are loaded with omega-3 fatty acids, substances that appear to reduce cholesterol and triglycerides in the blood, reduce the swelling from rheumatoid arthritis and prevent the blood clots that can trigger a heart attack or stroke.

In some people with migraine headaches, omega-3 fatty acids even seem to bring pain relief.

You can get these potent nutrients from supplements or from fatty fish. Plan two or three seafood meals each week and include fish such as Atlantic mackerel, salmon (pink or chinook), lake trout, whitefish, herring and anchovies.

284. Make a Healthy Soup

Soup not only tastes "mmm-mmm-good," it can keep you healthy, too.

The vegetables, beans and rice in some soups give you the fiber you need in your diet. Chicken soup helps relieve stuffy noses. Vegetable soup is packed with almost every vitamin that you need.

If you add a little bit of chicken to a vegetable soup or vegetables to a chicken soup, you enhance the health-promoting qualities of soup even more. The protein in chicken, along with the carbohydrates and fiber in vegetables, makes homemade soup almost a perfect meal. In addition, some studies show that eating a cup of soup before a main course can even help you lose weight.

There's something reassuring about a bowl of hot soup, no matter how you slurp it.

285. Fight the "Big C" with Vitamin C

No researchers claim that vitamin C alone can cure cancer. But the American Cancer Society recommends that you eat foods rich in vitamin C as part of an anti-cancer diet.

Studies at the Albert Einstein College of Medicine have shown that women with positive or suspicious Pap smears frequently have diets low in vitamin C. Vitamin C has also been shown in many studies to fight the viruses and toxins associated with cancer and other diseases.

If you don't think that you can get all the vitamin C you need from your diet, consider taking vitamin C supplements. There is little risk of overdose with this vitamin because excess amounts are quickly excreted in your urine.

Check with your doctor to see if some extra C is for you.

286. Learn to Survive Corporate Life

Barely a week goes by without another corporation announcing that it's downsizing. And although the adverse effects on the health of the people who are fired can be devastating, there can also be serious health consequences for the employees who remain.

After big layoffs, the employees who remain frequently have to handle more than their usual workloads. Here's what human resource and mental health experts say you should do to maintain your health if you're one of those left behind.

First, simplify life away from the job. Make more time for yourself and your family and friends. Second, even if you're working long hours, keep to your regular sleep schedule and get enough Zs. Third, eat a healthy breakfast and two other balanced meals every day. Fourth, and maybe most importantly, be good to yourself. Reward yourself with something positive and special each week.

And think about the future.

It can't hurt to send out feelers to see what opportunities may exist in a less stressful work environment.

287. Keep the Doctor Away with Herbs

Many people believe that there are alternatives to over-the-counter medications that can be used to fight cold and flu symptoms.

Echinacea angustifolia is one of the herbs most widely used to enhance the immune system. It has been shown to raise properdin levels. Properdin is a serum protein that naturally activates some of your body's defense mechanisms to fight infection. In addition, research shows that the herb stimulates your immune system. It helps your body produce a powerful disease-fighting chemical called interferon.

Next time you have the sniffles, reach for *Echinacea angustifolia* instead of your usual cold medicine. You can buy it at most health food stores and even at many pharmacies. It is available as a fresh, freeze-dried or dried herb and in liquid form. For more information, call the Herb Research Foundation in Boulder, Colorado, at 303-449-2265.

288. Sleep Like a Baby

If you are having trouble sleeping, you may not be thrilled at the idea of resorting to prescription or over-the-counter sleep aids. Perhaps you have even tried drugs to help you sleep, but they haven't worked. You may have even tried herbal remedies, meditation and relaxation exercises but still find yourself lying in bed at night staring at the ceiling, unable to sleep. You wish you could just sleep like a baby—and that may be the precise answer to your problem!

You may be sleeping in the wrong position. A fitness expert at the Massachusetts Institute of Technology suggests that you sleep in the fetal position. Instead of lying on your back or stomach, go to sleep on your side, knees bent at right angles to your body.

You may find that the secret to sleeping like a baby is simply to sleep like a baby.

289. Treat Morning Sickness Gingerly

Ginger can reduce the nausea and vomiting of morning sickness. It helps remove intestinal gas and relaxes the intestinal tract.

In one study, gingerroot powder significantly reduced the number of vomiting attacks and the severity of nausea and vomiting among women with even the worst morning sickness. The study used 250 milligrams of gingerroot powder four times a day to achieve these results.

Of course, no pregnant woman should use any substance as a drug without first discussing it with her doctor. But you may find that fresh gingerroot, which is available at most grocery stores, provides even better results. Just grate it into a batch of gingerbread cookies and enjoy!

290. Talk about Sex

In the past, it was falsely believed that seniors have no interest in sex, except for a few "dirty old men." A more current myth is that seniors are (or should be) highly sexually active.

Actually, your sexuality is in a constant state of change. As men get older, some take longer to achieve erection and orgasm. And some women experience a gradual decrease in sexual desire, while others become more sexually responsive. Menopause symptoms, illness and the normal effects of aging all contribute to your changing sexuality.

Surveys show that among seniors, sexual activity is more common than abstinence. And many married people over age sixty-five (even some in their eighties and nineties) still have sex regularly.

If you're experiencing sexual problems, talk to your doctor no matter what age you are. Whether your problem has a physical or an emotional cause, a few tips from your doctor may help you enjoy a satisfying sexual life.

291. Consider Hormone Replacement Therapy

You can get relief from the discomforts of menopause through hormone replacement therapy (HRT).

About 80 percent of women suffer hot flashes, night sweats, insomnia, depression and other symptoms that are associated with menopause.

With HRT, you are given small doses of the hormones estrogen and progesterone, which not only can relieve these symptoms but can help reduce vaginal dryness and prevent osteoporosis and heart disease as well. There is a small increase in the risk of endometrial and breast cancers with HRT. So if you have a personal or family history of cancer, or if you have high blood pressure, extreme obesity, liver disease, thrombophlebitis, a cholesterol lipid disorder or coronary artery disease, HRT is probably not for you.

If you do not have these health problems, however, HRT may do wonders for you. Good nutrition, regular exercise, stress management, calcium supplements, vaginal lubricants and other lifestyle choices can also help alleviate the symptoms of menopause.

292. Get Help for Cancer from Those Who Care

In 1994, about 750,000 people were helped by the service and rehabilitation programs of the American Cancer Society. The society has trained volunteers who provide transportation to and from treatment, and the society offers supplies and equipment to help at home.

You and your family can benefit from cancer support programs such as "I Can Cope" and from group programs for patients, families and friends.

Among the successful rehabilitation programs that the society provides are:

- "Reach to Recovery," for women with breast cancer

- "Laryngectomy Rehabilitation," run in collaboration with the International Association of Laryngectomies
- "Look Good, Feel Better," run in partnership with the National Cosmetology Association and Cosmetic, Toiletry and Fragrance Association
- "Can Surmount," a short-term support program for patients and families

There are also other useful programs for both children and adults who have cancer. Call your local unit of the American Cancer Society for more information. You can get the phone number from your local phone book.

293. Stand Up for Your Right to Healthy Air

Eliminate environmental tobacco smoke (ETS) where you live, work and play and reap the health benefits.

In December of 1992, the Environmental Protection Agency called ETS a "serious and substantial" health problem. Every year, about 3,000 nonsmoking adults die from disease caused by breathing other people's tobacco smoke. And that's not all. ETS causes 35,000–40,000 deaths from heart disease among nonsmokers. It can also aggravate conditions such as asthma, poor blood circulation, bronchitis and pneumonia.

The unborn fetus and young children also suffer from exposure to ETS. Children exposed to secondhand smoke experience more respiratory problems, while infants of mothers who smoke have a higher rate of sudden infant death syndrome.

Protect your health. Thank people for not smoking around you—wherever you may be. And ask those who do smoke around you to stop. The smoker's right to smoke stops when his or her smoke gets into the air you breathe.

294. Detect Cancer at a Curable Stage

The American Cancer Society has recommendations for the early detection of cancer in people without any obvious symptoms.

If you are between eighteen and thirty-nine years of age, you should probably have a cancer-related checkup every three years. The checkup should include an examination of the thyroid, mouth, skin and lymph nodes, as well as the testicles for men and the breasts, uterus, cervix and ovaries for women.

If you are age forty or over, your annual cancer checkup should include all of the above, plus colon and rectal examinations. Women should have a mammogram, and once over fifty, men should have a prostate exam.

These tests can help detect cancer early, at a more curable stage.

295. Choose to Be Happy

You can choose to be happy.

There's a saying you can use to help you change what you believe: "You can't change the wind, but you can adjust your sails." In other words, you can learn to respond to life's travails in a way that meets your needs. You can't change what happens, but you can change how you react to events.

Cognitive therapists have shown that most of us have "learned helplessness"—that is, we come to expect disappointment, rejection and so on. But these researchers have also proved that we can learn optimism. We can learn to change our thinking patterns. According to researchers at San Francisco's Saybrook Institute, it may not be as important to know how you reached your current state of health as it is to understand that you can take control of your own health—now!

And two books, readily available at libraries and bookstores, can get you started. One is *Healing from Within* by Dennis T. Jaffe, Ph.D.; the other, *Learned Optimism* by Martin E. Seligman, Ph.D.

296. Run from the Radura

Pay attention to the strange new symbol that is appearing on foods all over America. It's called the Radura, and it means that the foods have been irradiated.

The Food and Drug Administration has approved the irradiation of foods to help preserve them. This technique kills the bacteria that grow on a food and cause the food to spoil. Those in favor of food irradiation claim that it is safe and that it reduces the need for chemical preservatives to keep foods fresh longer.

Those who oppose irradiating fruits and vegetables, such as the New York Public Interest Research Group, say that irradiated foods may contribute to the development of cancer and other diseases, that irradiation destroys essential nutrients in foods, and that food irradiation plants themselves are hazardous to the employees and people who live nearby.

The final scientific answer isn't in on who's right, so you may want to pass up irradiated foods until it is.

297. Pinch Yourself!

Are you carrying too much fat? The pinch test will tell you the real story.

Pinch a fold of skin to the side of your stomach, halfway up the back of your thigh or on the upper part of your arm and measure it. All you need is an ordinary ruler. Every one-quarter inch of flesh above one inch equals ten pounds of extra fat. (One inch or less in the pinch test means that your body fat level is low or moderate.)

And don't think you shouldn't take the test because you're thin. You can look thin but still be fat when too high a percentage of your body weight is fat.

Try this test at home. The answer can help you head in the right direction.

298. Lose Weight Gradually

If you're trying to lose weight, do so gradually and you're more likely to keep it off.

Try to lose one-half to one pound a week, or two to three pounds in a month. Aim to attain a healthy weight a year from now, not next week.

Setting small, achievable goals for yourself will also keep you away from the crash diets and fad diets that inevitably lead to failure. Success breeds success, and you may soon achieve a weight goal that has eluded you for a long time.

299. Be a Healthy Shopper

Nutrition experts and consumer advocates recommend that you follow these six tips to be a healthy shopper.

1. Plan your healthy meals before you go shopping.
2. Write down what you need and take the list with you to the store.
3. Eat before you go to the supermarket. If you're hungry, you may not be able to resist fat-laden goodies.
4. Avoid aisles that are loaded with soft drinks, high-fat potato chips, candy, cake and ice cream.
5. Stick to the aisles that contain fresh fruits and vegetables, whole grains, beans and other ingredients on your list.
6. Be careful! Every smart consumer knows that the supermarkets place tempting items—which are not good for you—around the cash registers to seduce you while you wait in line.

300. Accentuate the Positive

Focusing on positive events that have occurred throughout the day can increase your health and even protect you from disease.

Sometimes it's hard to do that. Family problems, trouble at work and other daily hassles can color and cloud your day. But scientific research has shown that positive emotions produce positive biochemical responses in your body. And these complex biochemical processes play an important part in how you feel.

So when you get home each day, sit back and think of all the things that went right. Even better, get a pen and paper and write down the positive events of the day.

This simple action can reduce a great deal of stress, offset the effects of the day's negative events and give you something that everybody needs: perspective.

301. Worry for Thirty Minutes

Millions of Americans worry away long stretches of the day, reports the National Institute of Mental Health. And most worries are about things that never happen. Yet while people worry about what might happen—developing health problems related to anxiety along the way—life slips by unlived.

A Pennsylvania State University psychologist has developed a practical plan that can help you reduce the time you spend worrying. Among his suggestions are two that can free up a great deal of time for enjoying life. First, set aside thirty minutes a day for worrying. And second, write down a list of things to worry about during that period.

These two suggestions can be your first steps to limiting—and then eliminating—needless worry in your life.

302. Beat the Holiday Blues

Many people feel blue or depressed around the holidays, especially during the long stretch beginning with Thanksgiving and ending on New Year's Day. Unfortunately, holidays that should be full of cheer can sometimes highlight what you feel is lacking in your life, such as a loved one who has passed away.

But you can beat the holiday blues by being aggressive. If you're on your own, invite people to visit. And if an old holiday tradition, such as a big Thanksgiving dinner or breakfast on Christmas morning, brings back painful memories—start anew! Do something different this year. Just make sure you avoid alcohol. It's a depressant and can make you feel low.

Holidays are wonderful times to take the focus off yourself and help those who are needy. Remember, shelters and soup kitchens always need volunteers.

303. Know When to Fold

Are you a "heavy drinker" or an alcoholic? Some experts say that if you think you have a problem with alcohol, then you probably do.

Either way, if you feel that alcohol is playing too big a role in your life, talk to your doctor, a religious adviser or a counselor. There are many ways you can find help for a drinking problem. If you are too embarrassed to bring the subject up in person, call Alcoholics Anonymous. The number is in your local phone directory. And most hospitals, medical clinics and community service agencies have outpatient and inpatient alcohol treatment programs that can help you find your way out of a bottle.

304. Avoid Sleeping Pills

No one has ever died from a lack of sleep—but there have been deaths from the misuse of sleeping pills.

That's because even if you use prescription sleeping pills exactly as intended, you can get addicted. Or you can develop a tolerance for the pills and need to take more than you should to get the same results. Older people have a lower tolerance for medication than the young or middle-aged and need to be extra careful.

If you want to stop taking sleeping pills, wean yourself off them gradually. Quitting cold turkey can have serious health consequences.

If you're having trouble getting or staying asleep, talk to your doctor about nondrug approaches to insomnia that are safer than powerful pills.

305. Loosen Your Tie

Whether you still wear Eisenhower-era ties or sport a hip Jerry Garcia tie, that noose-like piece of apparel may be interfering with your vision.

Researchers at Cornell University have concluded that neckties that are knotted too tightly can block blood flow to the brain and eyes.

How tight is too tight?

Slip your finger between your neck and shirt collar. If it won't go in, the tie is too tight.

If you like to wear a necktie, make sure you buy shirts with enough room at the neck. Loosen your tie during the day and leave the top shirt button open. No one will see it under the knot in your tie.

306. Alleviate the Pain of Male Menopause

If you're a male between ages forty and sixty, you may go through emotional changes that some experts are calling male menopause. You may begin to feel pessimistic, overburdened, nervous and dissatisfied. Or you may have trouble sleeping, begin to abuse alcohol and/or drugs, become unhappy at work and at home, and develop sexual problems. You suddenly may even consider taking big risks with your life.

If you think you're undergoing male menopause, stay away from the "relief" offered by drugs and alcohol. Talk to your spouse and close friends. Sharing your feelings will ease the tension you feel. Don't make major changes impulsively, such as getting a divorce or quitting your job. Step back. And think things over.

If your problems persist, consider talking to a professional.

307. Go to Bed!

The number one sexual problem in America today affects people in their twenties, people in their fifties and everyone in between. It's called inhibited sexual desire (ISD).

Millions of Americans are too stressed out to do anything in bed but sleep. Financial worries, pressures at work and problems at home are having a negative effect on the love lives of millions of people in the prime of life.

One of the most important things a couple can do to weather ISD is to go to bed together, at the same time. Let any unfinished business go until tomorrow. If you don't feel like making love, you can still hug and kiss and cuddle.

Talk to your doctor if your sexual life doesn't regain its vigor. Other factors, such as medication or alcohol use, may be complicating the situation.

308. Take Snoring Seriously

Snoring may signal a life-threatening condition. If your partner's snoring ruins your sleep, the answer may not be separate bedrooms. Your partner may need to see a doctor.

People who snore loudly may suffer from sleep apnea, a condition in which the person stops breathing and has to gasp for air. Sleep apnea can be caused by enlarged tonsils or adenoids or by a disturbance of the central nervous system.

You need to take this condition seriously, because sleep apnea can sometimes bring on a stroke or heart attack.

Most people with sleep apnea are overweight. Alcohol and sleeping pills can make the condition worse.

If someone has told you that you snore loudly, see your doctor. You don't want to take this problem lightly.

309. See the Eye Doctor and Keep Your Vision Sharp

You can help fend off an attack of macular degeneration, the most common cause of legal blindness in the United States today. With this condition, the central area of the retina deteriorates. As a result, you lose central vision.

Macular degeneration is a disease that most frequently affects the elderly. Blurred vision is its main symptom. You may also begin to have difficulty reading fine print and seeing distant objects, although peripheral (side) vision is fine.

Regular eye exams will help catch the disease, and doctors are now having success treating—and slowing the progress of—this disease with laser therapy.

But early diagnosis is the key to successful treatment. And early diagnosis depends on seeing your ophthalmologist.

310. Don't Be So Sweet

If you're an average American, you eat 125 pounds of sugar a year—much of it unconsciously. That's because about 75 percent of the sugar you eat is added to foods before you ever see it: Ketchup, soups, salad dressings, canned and frozen fruits and vegetables, juices and many other food items contain sugar.

Nutritionists disagree on sugar in the diet. Some believe sugar is okay if you have a healthy diet, while others think it contributes to cavities and diseases such as obesity, diabetes, high blood cholesterol and hypertension.

While the debate goes on, you can substitute fresh fruits for sugary snacks and get carbohydrates from healthy foods instead of "empty calories" from sugar.

311. Fight Intolerance

People who are lactose-intolerant are unable to digest milk and milk products. Gas, diarrhea, abdominal cramps, bloating and other uncomfortable symptoms can appear within a few hours of drinking milk or eating milk products.

Many people outgrow their need for milk and milk products, and their bodies develop a deficiency in the enzyme needed to digest milk. This problem is more common among women because they drink more milk than men to keep their calcium levels high.

Lactose intolerance is not an all-or-nothing thing. If you're lactose-intolerant, you can still have small amounts of milk. And even if you're highly sensitive, you can add Lactaid (sold in liquid and tablet forms) to milk, which will provide the missing enzyme. Or you can drink soy milk or milk already treated with lactose.

Although lactose intolerance is usually not a serious problem, see your doctor if symptoms persist to be sure you don't have a more serious disorder.

312. Prevent Food Poisoning

Most food poisoning causes only minor problems that disappear quickly. But you must be careful, because the toxic agents that cause these problems can occasionally prove fatal.

If you experience severe stomach cramps, diarrhea and vomiting a few hours after eating, you probably have a case of food poisoning. Most often bacteria have contaminated food that was improperly handled. Less often food poisoning is caused by eating a food that is actually poisonous, such as a toxic mushroom.

Don't try to stop the vomiting or diarrhea. This is how your body is getting rid of the poison. To prevent dehydration, drink small amounts of water at frequent intervals.

If symptoms persist or worsen, or if there is blood in the vomit or diarrhea, call your doctor immediately.

Protect yourself from food poisoning by being scrupulous about cleanliness in the kitchen—wash your hands, wash all foods before cooking and cook foods thoroughly.

313. Check Dizziness with Your Doctor

People with low blood pressure have great life expectancies, but they can sometimes faint during intense emotional experiences. And after severe injuries, blood pressure can drop to dangerously low levels that lead to shock.

Low blood pressure can be caused by genetics, dehydration, medications, chronic anxiety, tension or glands that are out of whack. If you find yourself feeling dizzy or occasionally faint, see your doctor to rule out any serious underlying condition.

314. Protect Yourself from Carpal Tunnel Syndrome

Carpal tunnel syndrome is affecting increasing numbers of people who perform repetitive work with their hands. Meat cutters, assembly line workers and those who use keyboards are at particular risk.

The carpals are small bones in the wrist. Along with ligaments just beneath the skin, they form a tunnel. A nerve passes through this tunnel, sending signals to the fingers and thumb. So if swelling or inflammation occurs in this area, the ligaments may press on the nerve, giving you pain, tingling or numbness in your fingers and a shooting pain in your wrist and arm. This condition can become severe, serious and chronic.

You can prevent carpal tunnel syndrome by minimizing the stress on your wrists and fingers. Take frequent breaks from any repetitive task, and perform hand exercises to relax the muscles and improve circulation. Over-the-counter anti-inflammatory drugs can help reduce symptoms. You may even want to consider using wrist splints, which should be fitted by your doctor.

315. Eat for Your Teeth

Nutritional research shows that a balanced diet of dairy products, poultry, fish, vegetables, fruits and whole grains is essential for healthy teeth and gums.

What's more, eating raw, crunchy vegetables stimulates your gums and helps clean your teeth. That's why some dentists call vegetables such as broccoli and cauliflower detergent vegetables.

Next time you go food shopping, make sure these "detergents" are on your list. What you eat—and what you don't eat—can affect whether you keep or lose your teeth as you age.

316. Treat Dentures Naturally

It's as important to take care of your dentures as it is to take care of your natural teeth.

Plaque builds up on false teeth just as it does on normal teeth. It can not only cause mouth odors but also irritate the soft tissues of your mouth.

That's why you should brush your dentures every day. You can use baking soda as a cleaner, although many people find that it's not as effective as commercial denture cleaners. Do not use bleach. It fades the color of your dentures, tarnishes metal parts and burns your mouth.

You may have lost your natural teeth, but with good oral hygiene, you can still have a winning smile.

317. Zap Plaque

Periodontal disease, or pyorrhea, can lead to the destruction of the bone around the roots of your teeth, which will cause them to loosen and fall out. It affects nine out of ten adults and is the major cause of tooth loss in people over age forty.

The key to preventing this disease is removing plaque, a sticky, invisible film that builds up on teeth. You can see the plaque on your teeth if you chew a disclosing tablet which contains a harmless dye that turns plaque red. After you chew the tablet, rinse your mouth. The areas of plaque will be bright red. You can then brush and floss, paying extra attention to the areas of plaque. After you brush, rinse out your mouth. If the red remains, brush and floss one more time.

Disclosing tablets are available from your local pharmacy.

318. Let Go of That Strong Jaw

If you have temporomandibular disorder (TMD), you will usually feel pain on the upper cheek, about three-quarters of an inch in from the center of your ear. With this condition, the jaw muscles, joints and ligaments are out of place. As a result, your jaw may make snapping sounds when you move it, and you may get headaches on the side where your jaw hurts. People with TMD also tend to grind their teeth at night.

Help yourself by learning to notice when you clench your jaw or grind your teeth. Ask your spouse or friends to tell you when they notice you clenching your jaw or grinding your teeth. Make a conscious effort to relax your jaw when you become aware of the tension there.

You can help minimize TMD by exercising regularly (this relieves tension overall) and by adding more enjoyment to your life. Short-term psychotherapy can help, too, by helping you learn to cope better with stress through relaxation techniques and changes in attitude.

319. Beat Fatigue

Fatigue sends more than ten million Americans to their doctors each year.

If you're eating well and getting enough sleep, exercise may be able to eliminate fatigue and boost your energy—especially if you have a job that keeps you seated most of the day. What's more, exercise acts as a natural tranquilizer, relieving fatigue that may be caused by stress.

Next time you're feeling tired, get up and go out for a walk in the fresh air. Something as simple as this can re-energize you in a matter of minutes.

The Royal Canadian Exercise Plan is an excellent starting point if you haven't been exercising regularly. Only five to seven minutes with this plan each morning will get you energized and off to a vigorous day. Borrow a copy of the revised United States edition of the official *Royal Canadian Air Force Exercise Plans for Physical Fitness* from your local library. Or buy your own copy from your neighborhood bookstore.

320. Protect Your Vocal Cords

Most of us don't think about our vocal cords until we develop laryngitis or become hoarse. But like any other tissue, your vocal cords can become strained through overuse.

You can help protect your voice by keeping the air in your home from getting too dry. Also, make sure to drink eight to ten glasses of water each day, and your vocal cords will get the lubrication they need.

Speak softly if you need to be on the telephone for long periods of time. Use a headset or phone rest, too. Muscle tension in the face, neck and throat can increase tension in the vocal cords. And try not to speak in a tone of voice that is higher or lower than your normal pitch. This causes strain.

If you become hoarse despite these precautions, don't whisper. Whispering requires more effort than speaking softly. And avoid speaking at all unless you absolutely must.

321. Microwave Safely

Microwaves are convenient, but bacteria can grow in microwave-cooked foods because these devices cook foods unevenly. Although food cooks quickly, some parts of the food may not be cooked at all. Bacteria and other microorganisms in the uncooked portions can then cause food poisoning.

To prevent this from happening, always thaw meats before cooking them in the microwave. Cover the cooking vessel you use with a lid or with plastic wrap made for use in microwaves. This will trap steam and help cook the food properly. Leave the lid slightly ajar or poke a hole in the plastic wrap to allow ventilation. When you remove food from the microwave, let it stand. The food will continue to cook for several minutes.

322. Avoid Tanning Salons

Tanning is a sign of damage to the skin. Thirty minutes in a tanning salon is like two to three hours in the midday sun—and experts from all over the world warn that regular exposure can wrinkle your skin and trigger skin cancer.

Researchers from the American Academy of Dermatology have found that exposure to UVA and UVB rays at tanning salons also suppresses your body's immune system, causes cells to swell and is hazardous to your sight. Studies have shown that exposure to UVB rays is linked with cataracts and retinitis. And the rays can react with soaps and cosmetics you use, damaging your skin and causing rashes.

To top it all off, very few states regulate tanning salons, increasing the dangers they present to you. Do yourself a favor and avoid tanning salons. You may want to try some of the newer sunless tanning lotions now available. Just don't forget to use a sunscreen over your tanning lotion when you're out in the sun.

323. Turn Down the Volume

You may be so used to the noise in your environment that you don't even know how loud it is anymore.

The United States government estimates that 10 percent of Americans are exposed to such extreme levels of noise for long-enough periods of time that permanent hearing loss results.

Some things are beyond your control, such as air traffic and street construction, but there are things you can do to protect your hearing.

If you listen to music on earphones, don't turn the volume up to block out external sounds. At home or in the car, play the stereo at moderate volume. If you live on a noisy street, use double drapes to absorb outside sounds. And don't be ashamed or too self-conscious to wear earplugs anywhere there's too much noise.

324. Tell Your Story

Give yourself some time each day to record what you've seen, heard and felt during your time here on earth. Write about your feelings and reflections.

Most of us love stories of all kinds: adventure, romance, thrillers, mysteries and so on. We love fiction and true-life tales. And there are great rewards to be gained from reading.

But you can also benefit from telling your own story. Research shows that expressing your feelings in writing can help relieve stress from worry and even help you solve problems. Sometimes writing things down allows painful feelings to break through. Getting these feelings out can be beneficial physically and mentally.

325. Tailor Your Desk to Fit

Prevent problems for yourself by arranging your work area so that it suits your health needs.

You can reduce or even prevent back, neck and leg pain by making sure your desk at home and on the job is at the right height.

How can you tell if it is?

When seated at your desk, your feet should be able to rest comfortably on the floor. Your desk should be seven to twelve inches above the seat of your chair. If you work at a keyboard, it should be at elbow level when you're sitting. And you should not have to lean forward to work at your desk. This will put unnecessary strain on your neck and back. Instead, try to keep your shoulders relaxed and your head in line with your spine.

Paying attention to these little details can pay off by preventing a great deal of pain and discomfort.

326. Learn the Heimlich Hug

You can dislodge an object from the throat of someone who is choking by using the Heimlich maneuver. If a person can't talk and grasps his or her throat, here's what you do.

1. Stand behind the person.
2. Wrap your arms around the person between the rib cage and navel.
3. Make a fist with one hand, putting the thumb against the person's abdomen.
4. Ask a conscious person to put his or her head upright.
5. Hold your fist with your other hand and quickly thrust upward into the person's abdomen four times. The thrusts must be powerful to dislodge the object causing the choking. If you don't succeed at first, immediately do it again.

The Heimlich maneuver is effective for almost everyone. It is not meant for children younger than one year. If you have an infant, ask your pediatrician to teach you what to do if your baby is choking.

327. Learn CPR

You can get blood flowing back to the brain of someone who has had a heart attack, drug overdose or electrical shock or who has stopped breathing for another reason by using cardiopulmonary resuscitation (CPR).

The basic procedure involves three steps.

1. Tilt the victim's head back to clear the airways.
2. Pinch the victim's nose and perform mouth-to-mouth resuscitation.
3. Use both hands to compress the heart and get blood circulating by pushing down at the midpoint of the front of the rib cage.

You can learn CPR in as little as three hours, but you need to learn it from an expert. Call your local chapter of the American Red Cross or the American Heart Association and ask about classes in CPR. Many local hospitals teach CPR as well.

328. Outfit Your Car for Survival

You never know what can happen on a car trip, so make sure your car is equipped with a survival kit.

Your kit should include a complete first aid kit, matches, flares and a white cloth to signal distress. It should include water, food, a flashlight with extra batteries, a small fire extinguisher and a knife. You should also carry an empty gas can and change for phone calls.

And don't forget to add items as the seasons change. A snow shovel, chains for the wheels, blankets, and sand or gravel (to put under the tires in case you get stuck on ice or in mud) should be added during cold weather.

329. Shovel Snow Safely

Almost everyone knows that shoveling snow can be risky, but people do it anyway. If you are over forty, are overweight, have high blood pressure, smoke or lead an inactive life, you probably shouldn't try to shovel snow. You may have an undiagnosed heart condition that could flare up under the stress of snow shoveling. Talk to your doctor and see what he or she advises you to do.

If you absolutely must shovel snow, dress in several warm layers of clothes. And be careful with the amount of snow you shovel. Don't fill the blade with snow, especially when it's a heavy, wet snow. Move smaller amounts.

If possible, find someone with a snowblower or a teenager who wants to earn some money. The job will be done more quickly—and you won't be in any danger.

330. Give Your Doctor All the Facts

A survey at Harvard University revealed that most doctors think they spend more than ten minutes talking and listening to their patients during appointments. The researchers found that in reality, doctors spend less than two minutes.

Since your doctor may not be taking the time to get all the information he needs to help you make decisions related to your health, take the initiative. Tell your physician about the things you think are important.

For example, let your doctor know if you live alone, eat a lot of junk food or feel stressed out. Tell him about your job and any toxic substances you may be exposed to at work. Tell him if and how much you exercise, drink or smoke. And talk about your feelings and emotional life. Is your sex life satisfying? Are you thinking of divorce? Are you worried about your kids?

Your doctor needs a complete picture of everything in your life that could conceivably affect your mental and physical functioning.

Otherwise, recommended treatment for various problems that arise may be ineffective.

331. Carry the Card—A Health ID Card

A health ID card can save your life.

If you're in an accident, or if you have a heart attack, you may not be able to communicate with the medical people assisting you. Or you may be injured in another country and not speak the language.

That's why it's extremely important to carry a medical ID card if you have a condition that can require emergency medical attention, such as diabetes. You can get a Medic Alert tag by calling the Medic Alert Foundation at 1-800-344-3226 or by writing to them at P.O. Box 1009, Turlock, CA 95831. In addition, many HMOs provide cards on which you can write important health information. And some hospitals offer complete medical histories on small microfiche cards that you can carry with you.

332. Get a Fire Extinguisher

Smoke detectors aren't enough to protect your family from fire. Get a home fire extinguisher and learn how to use it. Your home should have at least one fire extinguisher, mounted in plain view, out of a child's reach and easy-to-use.

Fire extinguishers are made for different purposes. Your best bet is to get a multipurpose extinguisher. Look for one with a rating of 2A10BC or higher. You can also tell if a product is safe by looking for the Underwriter's Laboratories (UL) or Fire Mutual (FM) code of approval.

Look at the directions and make sure that you understand them fully before buying the product. And once you get the extinguisher home, make sure you check the pressure indicator monthly to be sure the device is working.

333. Move Fast When Poison Is Involved

Don't panic but get moving if you think you or a member of your household has swallowed something poisonous, gotten poisonous material in the eyes or absorbed by the skin, or inhaled poisonous fumes or vapors.

Call your local Poison Control Center immediately. (You should have this number posted by the phone.) Or call your doctor or local hospital. Explain what happened as simply and clearly as you can. If possible, identify the poison.

You can handle most cases of poisoning at home. But you must remain calm, so you can listen to the instructions you receive and follow them exactly.

You should always keep a bottle of syrup of ipecac and a bottle of activated charcoal in your medicine cabinet. The ipecac induces vomiting, while the charcoal absorbs poison. Depending on the type of poison that has been ingested, your Poison Control Center may suggest you use one or the other.

334. Feast on Fiber

Most everyone these days is trying to increase the amount of fiber they eat. If you find it difficult to get enough fiber, try these five easy ways to get what you need.

- Get whole grains from breakfast cereals. Or if you can't seem to do that, try corn tortillas, brown rice, whole-wheat pasta or bulgur wheat at lunch or dinner.
- Eat strawberries, raspberries, blackberries and other fruits with seeds.
- Eat vegetables that have edible stems, such as broccoli.
- When possible, eat the skins of potatoes and other vegetables.
- Always eat whole-wheat and other whole-grain breads.

Follow these five easy pieces of advice, and you'll get the fiber you need.

335. Hurry-up Slow-Cooking Healthy Foods

Some high-fiber foods may take too long to cook in the traditional way to accommodate your schedule. But you can keep them in your diet by zapping them in your microwave.

Artichokes can take up to forty-five minutes to cook the standard way, but covered loosely and put in the microwave at full power, they can be ready to eat in only five minutes. And eggplant, which can take an hour or more to cook in an oven, can be on your plate after only seven minutes in the microwave.

Be creative and see what other kinds of healthy foods can be prepared with less bother and in less time using a microwave oven.

336. Heal Yourself through Gardening

Grow your own healthy foods or beautiful flowers, and you'll grow healthier, too.

Researchers at the University of Delaware have found that people respond to plants in the environment with lowered blood pressure, reductions in heart rate and relaxation of muscle tension.

People actively involved in gardening benefit even more from that activity because gardening keeps them limber and keeps their muscles toned. It does wonders for stress. And anyone can grow healthy foods that will help fight disease.

Gardening is the number one outdoor leisure activity in the United States. Maybe you should try it.

337. Get Out of Yourself and Into a Book

Reading can help relieve a great deal of stress and tension. It can get you "out of your head" and away from many self-centered fears and worries. It can provide a welcome escape from difficult situations and relax you from head to toe.

Whether you read romance novels, history books or books on

nature or astronomy, pick one up today and read for thirty minutes. And don't say you don't have time. Even the late president John F. Kennedy enjoyed reading James Bond novels.

Whatever you read, you'll find the activity relaxing, rewarding and enriching. And it is almost certain that you will feel more mentally alert after reading for an hour or two than after sitting and staring at a TV for the same length of time. TV engages your eyeballs. A book engages your mind.

338. Use Ginger for Motion Sickness

In a recent study of individuals who experience motion sickness, scientists tested the old motion sickness remedy Dramamine against a placebo and gingerroot powder. The participants were divided into three groups, given a capsule with one of the substances, and then sent rocking and rolling in a revolving chair.

The results showed that powdered gingerroot was the most effective substance in reducing motion sickness symptoms. So next time you find the earth moving in odd ways, talk to your doctor about the usefulness of ginger for controlling motion sickness.

339. Try Music for Migraines

Music can tame the savage beast, soothe your soul and—so it seems—reduce migraine pain.

A researcher at California State University unexpectedly found that one group of people participating in a study experienced less migraine headache pain when they listened to music than did other participants in the study who did not listen to music.

According to the researcher, the frequency of headaches in the music group dropped threefold. The psychologist theorized that the soothing sounds reinforced what the participants learned from relaxation and visualization techniques.

See if music also helps reduce the intensity of your migraines.

340. Ask Your Airline to Help You Breathe

If you have respiratory problems, airlines are happy to make your trips easier if you let them know ahead of time when you'll be traveling.

The cabin pressure in most airplanes is lower than on the ground at sea level, for example. So if you have any respiratory problem such as emphysema, bronchitis or asthma, test your breathing before flying. Walk 100-200 feet without stopping. If you have trouble, ask your airline to provide oxygen for you on the flight. You will need a written letter from your doctor, and there will be a fee for the service, but it can make the difference between having a wonderful trip and enduring a distressful flight.

Airlines are also willing to help people with other health problems fly safely. Talk to your doctor and your travel agent.

341. Stay Alert at the Wheel

According to the National Traffic Safety Commission, "highway hypnosis" frequently occurs on long trips during which the scenery rarely changes. You can fall into a trance from staring straight ahead at the road. You won't be able to gauge your speed, and in extreme cases, you may even begin to hallucinate.

To prevent this from happening, keep your eyes moving. Don't just look straight ahead. Regularly check your rearview mirror and your side-view mirrors. Do this even if there isn't another car in view. You can also prevent highway hypnosis by shifting your point of focus. Look up the road seventy-five feet, then shift your focus to the dashboard, then back to the road.

If your eyes burn or you realize a period of time has gone by and you can't account for it, pull over. You've had enough driving.

342. Lend an Ear, Offer a Shoulder

When someone is recently bereaved, he often needs to express his feelings to get relief from his pain. And to help, all you have to do is listen.

Most bereavement counselors recommend that you let the bereaved do the talking. Just your being there—to hold hands or give a hug—helps him heal. Sometimes you won't say anything. You may just cry when the bereaved person cries.

You can also help by volunteering to do small chores around the house or to go shopping or do other errands. Remember to invite the bereaved person to come over to your place or to go out for a meal in the weeks and months after his loss.

As time goes on, family and friends return to their normal routines. This is when you can really be there for someone who has lost a loved one.

343. Retreat to Move Ahead

To move on after a broken marriage or relationship, you may first need to retreat. And one retreat that is guaranteed to fight off the negative health effects of sadness is a health spa. In fact, a trip to a health spa may be what you need to begin healing.

Spas are not just for the rich and famous. There are many wonderful—and affordable—spas across the country. And some offer special weekend or weeklong programs for the brokenhearted.

Participants attend seminars on self-esteem, learn relaxation techniques, eat well, exercise and enjoy recreational activities.

There are many excellent books in the library and in bookstores on spas and the special programs they offer. Your travel agent can also be of assistance in helping you choose a spa—and maybe in getting you a good deal as well!

344. Skate Away the Blues

Gray, leaden skies and long periods of freezing temperatures can get you down. And according to a psychologist at the Medical College of Pennsylvania, your self-esteem can plummet with the mercury during winter months, when you spend too much time indoors.

The psychologist recommends that you fight winter blues by reaching out and getting out. Call some friends and ask them to go skating with you, either outdoors or at a skating rink.

Get yourself a bright red scarf and a colorful matching cap to balance the gray of winter. The sunlight and physical activity will give you a lift and start your body pumping out endorphins, nature's mood enhancers.

When cold weather comes, don't hibernate. Get active and beat the winter blues.

345. Live Out Your Deepest Dream

The next time you're alone, sit back and relax. Then think: Is there something you've always wanted to do but put off for one reason or another?

Almost everyone has a dream that has been denied, whether it's to finish college, go to Paris, return to the birthplace of your parents, learn to play the piano, study acting or take up painting. And now may be just the time to do it or to lay the groundwork for making that dream come true.

A deep dream finally lived out can renew the life force in you and do more for your health, appearance and self-esteem than any drug, technique or cosmetic ever could.

You may need to save money or get more information, or you may be able to take action right now. Whatever the situation, make your dream come true—and enjoy the benefits that come to you.

346. Keep the Romance Alive

Couples who have been together for decades say that all it takes to keep love alive is a little effort.

You may find that "rituals" help recapture special feelings. Return regularly to a place that played an important role in your love, such as the spot where you decided to marry or where you spent your honeymoon.

Others find rejuvenation in trying things they've never done before—spending a weekend in the city, surprising one another with dinner and dancing, or even going to another country—to celebrate their love.

According to Robert N. Butler, M.D., of Mount Sinai Medical Center in New York City, some people go to bed together, hold each other in their arms and fall in love all over again.

The greatest pleasure in learning the secrets of lasting love is the process of learning itself.

347. Pat, Purr and Play with Your Pet

They help relieve pain, reduce tension, lower blood pressure and combat depression. They are recommended by 50 percent of doctors and psychologists in the United States. And they are not a new class of wonder drugs. They are *pets*.

All across the country, researchers are documenting the great health benefits that pets bring to their owners. Dogs and cats top the list of favorite pets in America, but fish, birds, hamsters and many other animals can do the trick just as well. At the University of Pennsylvania, Aaron Katcher, Ph.D., and his colleagues have shown that pets do wonders for their owners. In one experiment, they showed that when an owner was with his pet, the owner's blood pressure dropped lower than when he was resting.

Remember, not all pets are for everyone—but you may find that the benefits of owning a pet far outweigh the burdens of responsibility.

348. Watch What You Eat during Ragweed Season

Ragweed season begins in August and lasts until November in most areas of America. September is usually the peak for the plant that triggers hay fever. But ragweed may not be to blame for your sneezing and wheezing. It may be what you're eating.

According to researchers at the Allergy and Asthma Research Center of the New Jersey Medical Center, up to 30 percent of hay fever sufferers have allergic cross-reactions to foods that increase their responses to plant allergens.

Cantaloupe, honeydew melons, watermelon and bananas are often the culprits, as are certain spices, such as anise, caraway, coriander, cumin, parsley and parsnip. And if you are sensitive to birch or mugwort pollen, then celery, carrots, apples, potatoes and peaches may increase your allergic reaction.

Take care of your allergies and watch what you eat when the pollen count is high.

349. Use Painkillers Sparingly

More than ten million Americans suffer from chronic tension headaches and use aspirin, acetaminophen, ibuprofen or naproxen sodium to treat their headaches. But these painkillers, called analgesics, can cause headaches themselves, say researchers at the New England Center for Headache.

That's because overuse of these drugs interferes with the body's own natural painkillers and causes rebound headaches. Rebound headaches are more likely to occur in people who take about five or six acetaminophen or aspirin tablets a day, but they have occurred in people taking only two pills a day.

If you suspect you're getting rebound headaches, talk to your doctor about gradually substituting other medication for the analgesics you're taking.

350. Exercise Your "Muscle of Love"

Yes, Virginia, there is a "love muscle." It's called the pubococcygeal muscle, and there is an exercise that can help both men and women strengthen it and enhance their sex lives.

According to a researcher at Loyola University of Chicago Stritch School of Medicine, the Kegel exercise strengthens the "love muscle" and allows men to make love longer (by preventing premature ejaculation). In women, the exercise apparently produces more satisfying orgasms.

In both men and women, the pubococcygeal muscle controls urination. You can strengthen it by contracting it as if you were preventing urination. Each morning, contract this muscle thirty-six times, then rest for two minutes. Contract the muscle another thirty-six times, then rest for another two minutes. Do this for ten minutes.

You can expect to see results after several weeks.

351. Take a Drink from the Fountain of Youth

Talk to your doctor about fighting aging and illness with dehydroepiandrosterone (DHEA) supplements. DHEA is a hormone your body produces that helps keep things running smoothly. It can enhance your overall sense of well-being and may even help protect you against medical problems associated with aging.

According to researchers at the the Center for Mind-Body Medicine in Washington, D.C., many studies in animals and human beings have shown evidence that DHEA offers a wide range of health benefits without major side effects. Among the conditions that DHEA may help to prevent—or even reverse—are heart disease, cancer, diabetes, osteoporosis, obesity, autoimmune disorders (such as AIDS, lupus and rheumatoid arthritis) and Alzheimer's disease. The data on this hormone are so positive that it may even be of benefit to anyone over age forty, not just to those with medical problems.

352. Check How You Feel before You Get Behind the Wheel

If you drive a car and are taking one of the 300,000 over-the-counter (OTC) drugs that are available, AAA (the national auto club) recommends that you see how you feel after taking the OTC before you get behind the wheel of your car.

OTC products are not harmless. In fact, many OTC drugs can pose as much of a danger to a driver as alcohol. Antihistamines, cough suppressants and decongestants, for example, can seriously impair your driving ability. These drugs can cause drowsiness, dizziness and/or blurred vision. They can also cause disorientation and severe anxiety.

If the Food and Drug Administration has decided that the ingredients in an OTC product can impair driving ability, there will be a warning label on the product. Always read the label of any OTC product carefully. If you have any questions, talk to the pharmacist. He or she will be more than happy to provide you with information about any drug that you're taking.

353. Take an Aspirin When You're Angry

If you have an "angry heart," taking an aspirin once a day may reduce the increased risk of heart attack that can come with outbursts of anger.

Researchers at Harvard Medical School and Deaconess Hospital in Boston studied more than 1,000 heart attack patients at dozens of medical centers in the United States. The researchers discovered that a healthy man has a 1 in 1 million chance of having a heart attack in any given hour. But within two hours of an angry outburst, that risk jumps to 2.3 in 1 million. Among "angry" patients who took aspirin regularly, the risk of heart attack was 1.4 times that of a healthy man. Among "angry" patients who did not take aspirin regularly, the risk was 2.9 times that of a healthy man.

(There were not enough women in the survey to allow the researchers to draw valid conclusions regarding women.)

Doctors don't yet understand the exact link between anger and heart attacks. But anger does increase the production of adrenaline (a stimulating hormone), increase the heart rate and raise blood pressure.

If you are prone to angry outbursts, ask your doctor if regular aspirin use can help reduce your heart attack risk.

354. Add Tomatoes to Your Diet

If you're a man, add tomatoes and tomato-based foods to your diet today. They can help protect you from prostate cancer.

Researchers at the Harvard School of Public Health recently studied the eating habits of 47,000 men and found that those who ate at least ten servings of tomatoes and tomato-based foods each week had a 45 percent reduction in the rate of prostate cancer. Men who ate four to seven servings of tomatoes and tomato-based foods each week had a 20-percent reduction in the rate of prostate cancer.

Why? Researchers don't know. They do know, however, that tomatoes are rich in the antioxidant lycopene and that tomatoes proved beneficial when eaten raw, in sauces, as juice and even cooked with pizza. The researchers recommend that you eat a variety of vegetables and aim for ten servings of tomatoes a week as part of your overall healthy diet.

355. Unload "Nocebos"

Take a good look at your beliefs and expectations today. You may be loading up on "nocebos" without even knowing it.

Your negative thoughts may be doing more harm to you than you think. Doctors have long been aware of the *placebo* effect: Patients get better in part because they believe they will improve.

Recently, a researcher at the federal Centers for Disease Control and Prevention reported on the *nocebo* effect: Patients with negative thinking can experience a wide range of health ailments, and possibly even die, all from their negative beliefs and expectations.

Many doctors are not yet aware of the nocebo effect and do not know that it can be fought with simple techniques such as more personal contact between the patient and doctor. You can help yourself by learning to redirect your thinking along more positive channels. *Learned Optimism* by Martin E. Seligman, Ph.D., is an excellent book that can teach you practical techniques to enhance the placebo effect and defuse the nocebo effect.

356. Wear Your Seat Belt

Make a habit of buckling your seat belt. It takes only a few seconds, and it could save your life.

Auto accidents are responsible for 30,000 deaths and 40,000 injuries per year, according to the National Highway Traffic Safety Administration, and are the leading cause of death for people ages six to thirty-three.

Studies show that those who did not wear safety belts and died as a result of being ejected would have lived and often would not have been seriously hurt had they remained in the car.

Another study indicated that safety belts can prevent head and neck injuries in rollovers 100 percent of the time.

In addition, one study found that motorists who used lap and shoulder belts in cars equipped with air bags had a 75 percent reduction in injuries and were 90 percent less likely to need intensive hospital care after a crash.

Forty-nine states now have laws requiring the use of seat belts. So buckle up—you'll be obeying the law and maybe even saving your life.

357. Give Natural Medicine a Chance

Maybe it's time to give naturopathic medicine a look. In early 1996, the conservative city council of King County, Washington, voted to establish the first government-subsidized natural medicine clinic in the United States. Council members themselves admitted using acupuncture, enzymes, vitamins, and botanical fluids to maintain and improve their own health.

The word *naturopathic* was coined by John Scheel in 1895 to describe a combination of many approaches to health, including nutrition and exercise, herbal medicine, homeopathy, hydrotherapy and other natural therapies. Belief in a "Life Force" and in the healing power of nature is central to naturopathic medicine.

Naturopaths believe disease is caused by toxic materials that accumulate in the body: an unhealthy diet, poor posture, negative emotions, potent drugs, alcohol, caffeine, tobacco, environmental contaminants and infectious microorganisms.

You can find licensed naturopathic doctors in the following states: Alaska, Arizona, Connecticut, Hawaii, Montana, Oregon and Washington.

358. Lighten Up On-Line

If you're having a tough day and need a good laugh, you can now find one on-line. Whether you're on a break on the job, working at a computer in your home or using a computer at your local library, you can lighten your load by logging on to one of the many "laff lines" now available on the Internet.

You can reach the Humor Project, for example, at the Internet address http://www.wizvax.net/humor/. A wealth of information on humor will be at your fingertips.

Do you enjoy Rodney Dangerfield?
Try http://www.rodney.com/rodney/index.html.

Do you like David Letterman?

He's at http://www.cbs.com/lateshow/ttlist.html.

Explore the world of Internet humor. It's fun for its own sake, and you'll find many styles of humor to brighten up your day.

359. Fly by Night

If you fly by night, you can eliminate much of the emotional stress and inconvenience of traveling by day.

There is less traffic to and from the airport, fewer delays, no long lines and less chance that your luggage will be lost. And there is another benefit: Fewer planes crash at night!

360. Enhance the Flavor of Life

When you have a choice, go for the real thing and pick the natural flavor over the artificial one. Eat a real strawberry instead of strawberry-flavored candy. Or drink real fruit juice instead of an artificially flavored, artificially colored "fruit" drink.

Experts worry that a whole generation of children is being raised on artificially flavored foods that have hundreds of calories and no nutritional value whatsoever. Eventually, these children will grow up to be malnourished adults, prone to infections, heart disease and cancer at a very early age if their habits don't change.

So be a good role model and do yourself a health-building favor as well: Pick natural flavors every time you get the chance.

361. Drink to Your Health

The 1995 Dietary Guidelines for Americans issued by the federal government acknowledge for the first time that you can raise a drink to your health. Moderate drinking may lower your risk of heart attack. The 1990 federal guidelines said drinking alcohol had no net health benefit.

The new guidelines do not encourage drinking, and they warn

of the dangers of drinking too much alcohol. The experts recommend moderate drinking for those who enjoy a glass of wine with dinner or a cocktail after work. Moderation is defined as no more than one drink a day for women and no more than two drinks a day for men. (The amounts recommended are based on average body weights.)

What counts as one drink? One twelve-ounce glass of regular beer, one five-ounce glass of wine and one and one-half ounces of eighty-proof distilled spirits each count as one drink.

The guidelines also note that a higher level of alcohol consumption can increase your risk of high blood pressure, stroke, heart disease, certain cancers, suicide, violent behavior and accidents. It is also recommended that children, adolescents, women who are pregnant or attempting to get pregnant and those taking medications not drink alcohol. And of course, don't drink if you're going to drive or if you know you have problems with alcohol.

362. Investigate Integral Medicine

Doctors who practice integral medicine believe that the mind and the body work together as a unit. They evaluate your health based on an examination of your whole life situation, not merely on looking at individual symptoms or the results of medical tests.

A doctor of integral medicine may prescribe an anti-inflammatory drug or an herbal tea. But the prescription will be based as much on who you are as on what symptoms you have.

Healing begins with you, and the goal in integral medicine is to help you live in harmony with nature. For more information, call the California Institute for Integral Studies at 415-753-6100.

363. Try Magnesium for Migraines

Magnesium deficiency can set the stage for migraines, and adding magnesium to your diet may prevent painful migraine attacks.

A number of researchers have uncovered a link between low magnesium levels and the onset of migraine headaches—and some cases of tension headache as well. Investigators found low levels of magnesium in the tissue of migraine patients. And supplementation has provided some relief.

If other approaches to controlling migraines aren't bringing relief, talk to your doctor about how magnesium might help you.

364. Learn Label Lingo

If you're trying to eat a more healthful diet, take some time to learn what the product labels can tell you.

The federal government has revamped the labels you find on food products to make them more up-to-date with today's health concerns and easier to read. Claims such as "low-fat" and "low-calorie" must now meet strict requirements enforced by the government. An ingredient list is now required on the labels of all foods with more than one ingredient. The side or back of a package must have a nutrition panel summarizing the product's nutritional information.

One new feature of the nutrition panel is the % Daily Values column. By using the % Daily Values, you can easily determine whether a food contributes a lot or a little of a particular nutrient. And you can compare different products with no need to do any calculations. Keep in mind that the % Daily Values are based on a 2,000-calorie-a-day diet.

To learn more about the new food label, call the Office of Food Labeling at 202-205-5229 or the Food and Drug Administration at 301-443-4166.

365. Go Where You've Never Gone Before

Hundreds of native New Yorkers have never been to the Empire State Building, the Statue of Liberty or Coney Island. And hundreds of San Franciscans have never walked across the Golden Gate Bridge.

No matter who you are or where you live, there's someplace you have promised yourself you'd go . . . someday. Make that someday *today*. Be spontaneous. Go yourself or pack your spouse and kids in the car and head out.

Visit a nearby lake, a park, a museum or just the old neighborhood you grew up in. Whatever the place, go there and enjoy the experience.

Being spontaneous adds to the pleasure of being alive. And it stimulates your body to produce chemicals that keep you healthy and vigorous.

Go where you've never gone before—and enjoy the journey.